The Afflicted Healer

With Body, Mind & Spirit Guest Authors

Mary Varga

No part of this publication may be reproduced, stored in a retrieval system, or transmitted in any form or by any means- electronic, mechanical, digital, photocopy, recording or any other—except for brief quotations in printed reviews, without the prior permission of the author.

The Afflicted Healer
Copyright © 2019 by Mary Varga.
All rights reserved.

Cover Design formatting by Lisa M. Prysock; front cover image and many other photos in this manuscript contributed by Peggy Harms Photography. Some photos contributed from the author's personal collection and others from the manuscript guest authors. Any graphics or illustrations are believed to be public domain unless otherwise noted.

Edited by J. Baker Hill.

To contact the publisher:
Lisa Prysock, 7318 Autumn Bent Way, Crestwood, Kentucky 40014, USA.

To contact the author:
Mary Varga, 2001 Lancashire Avenue, Unit 102, Louisville, Kentucky 40205, USA.

Links, websites, and addresses not guaranteed for the life of the book.

This is a work of biographical non-fiction with emphasis in physical, mental, and spiritual fitness. All contributing authors have granted their permission to Mary Varga in a release for their written portions and photo contributions for the express purpose of publication and promotion of the book. Author Mary Varga maintains a record of release from each author.

This work is cataloged in the Library of Congress.

Unless paraphrased or otherwise noted, all Scripture verses are taken from the Holy Bible, New International Version.

Dedication

This book is dedicated to all those who struggle with an affliction … whether it be of the body, the mind or the spirit. We all deal with obstacles in our life. This book was written to suggest different strategies to help manage them.

The Afflicted Healer is also dedicated to all of my guest authors whose contributions not only made the book possible, but filled it with different possibilities to help you live with your challenges. It has been a true joy to work with all of them, and very rewarding to see their desire to help readers with their knowledge. They may not be afflicted, but they are all healers.

Acknowledgments

Once again, the Holy Spirit prompted me to write this book, but it would not have happened without the hard work and excitement of my guest authors. I simply provided an outlet for them to share their knowledge and expertise with you.

A majority of the pictures in the book were provided by Peggy Harms Photography. I was amazed at Peggy's talent and ability to make her subjects feel comfortable and enjoy the picture-taking experience.

I want to again acknowledge Lisa Prysock, a friend and author, for handling all the nuts and bolts of the self-publishing process for me. Lisa IS my publisher!

My thanks go to Baptist Health Milestone for giving me free access to use their facility for picture-taking. Many of my guest authors are also therapists, trainers or instructors who work there.

Once again, J. Baker Hill provided excellent editorial work for not just my writing, but the writings of my 15 guest authors. That's a tall order!

Many thanks also to Michael Lattin, BMB Productions, for making an inspiring book trailer to help market my book.

Special thanks goes to Joe Sepanek for retrieving my manuscript from the recycle bin after I'd accidentally deleted it. Joe saved many months of work by many authors.

50% of online proceeds from my book will be given to the Brain Injury Alliance of Kentucky (BIAK). They have given me a name in the brain injury community. BIAK continues to provide help and support to all those affected by brain injury.

Table of Contents

Introduction

Be joyful in hope, patient in affliction, faithful in prayer.

Romans 12:12

This book is entitled *The Afflicted Healer* because that is one of the life roles that I have been honored and blessed to have for the past decade. I will explain my affliction, my healing and how I became a healer in the first three chapters. Then I will introduce other afflicted healers I've had the privilege of knowing in my life. These are the individuals called to help others in spite of, or even because of the challenges that they personally endure.

The rest of my book is devoted to different strategies for living an active life despite the challenges you may face. We ALL have afflictions, difficulties or challenges. Don't you? Some are temporary and some are life-long. Some are physical and others are emotional/mental.

Whether your affliction is of the body, the mind, or the spirit you will find guidance and direction in the chapters of this book. We all live with afflictions of some sort and we are not left alone to try to manage them. Healers are all around to lead, encourage & inspire us.

After my affliction, my brain injury, I rediscovered the love of family and friends I had left behind in Louisville, Kentucky, when I married and moved to Little Rock,

Arkansas. Through all my hardships, my faith in God naturally deepened, knowing that only He could get me through this tragedy.

Ironically, through my recovery, my passion for physical fitness never waned. Working out gave me a feeling of control over the deplorable conditions that had become my life. Eventually exercising, coupled with prayer and a lot of stubborn determination, brought me to a place of physical independence. I'm still slow as molasses but am able to do most things without needing assistance.

I always felt like "poor little Mary" as people helped me to do things that should've come naturally. I abhorred looking and feeling so needy. I dreamed of a day when I would be able to help someone again.

Then the Spirit moved me to achieve certifications in both Personal Training and Senior Fitness Instruction. That was the *aha* moment that led me on a journey of helping seniors maintain and improve their fitness level and thus, their independence. Since I struggled for so long to achieve my own physical independence after my traumatic brain injury, I believed God was calling me to offer my guidance and encouragement to others who were now, or could soon be, struggling with their own mobility and independence. I am now able to offer hope to others who may see their personal mobility starting to slip away.

My hope is that this book will give you some tools for maintaining personal independence and physical fitness, as well as spiritual and mental fitness for your journey. I spoke in *The Light Through My Tunnel* of how it took a village of family, friends and community to manage my new disabled life. It has taken a village of guest authors to compile *The Afflicted Healer*. I have called on numerous professionals (i.e. physicians, therapists, trainers ...) to encompass all the nuances of living an active and productive life despite various life challenges. I will begin each chapter with my own thoughts before turning the subject over to the professionals.

We are all tri-part beings ... spirit, mind and body. I believe all three are essential for living a peaceful, content life of purpose. In *The Light Through My Tunnel*, I show how having Christ as a daily part of my life improved it in ways I could only imagine. I will continue to begin each chapter with God's Word from the scriptures on the topic being discussed. I have also asked my local leader of Bible Study Fellowship (BSF) International, along with the pastor of my Catholic parish, to share their experiences in helping others turn their concerns over to the Lord for guidance and direction. That will address the spiritual element of our being.

I have included direction from a Life Coach and from a Christian counselor to speak about the mind element. How we think and what we think about will control everything else in our life! This mind element will also improve naturally with exercise. Use selfishness in a good way! By taking care of and improving your body, the sense of accomplishment and control will filter over to other areas of your life.

As for the body element, I encourage you to read on ... then get moving!

Chapter 1

The Affliction

For our light and momentary troubles are achieving for us an eternal glory that far outweighs them all.

2 Corinthians 4:17

In order to become an afflicted healer, it was necessary to suffer an affliction. My accident and my traumatic brain injury were my afflictions. I gave a very detailed description of my accident in my first book, *The Light Through My Tunnel.* It hasn't changed. So rather than reinventing the wheel, the following description is exactly what I wrote in my first book.

From *The Light Through My Tunnel:*

When the brain suffers a trauma like the one I had, it does not record a memory, and that is actually a blessing in disguise. *Thank You God*! This part of my story comes from facts I was told over and over again by my husband Drew or other family members. The feelings, however, I *do* remember.

It happened the day before my very first Mother's Day. I was looking forward to celebrating this special day for moms. Andrew was three months old already! We were expected at a cookout at Ben and Sherri Jo's house after the sailboat races. Drew was still at the sailing club. I stayed home to get myself and Andrew party-ready. When Drew finally arrived home, the party had already started. I left in a huff, taking 20-month-old Andrew with me. Drew would have to take his own car after he showered.

Ben and Sherri Jo lived just over a mile away. I drove through the neighborhood just beyond our house. As I began to accelerate again after stopping at a stop sign, a teenage boy barreled down the intersecting hill and T-boned my car. He did not have a stop sign, so technically, it was my fault. Today, that same intersection is a four-way stop. I have seen pictures of our damaged automobiles. I had just begun accelerating, so the boy must have been moving at a pretty good clip to cause our cars to be as crushed as they were.

Fortunately, I had worn my seat belt, so I was not thrown from the car. My brain ricocheted back and forth inside my skull, held in place by the seatbelt. I had only minor scrapes, with no cuts or broken bones. Andrew still slept safely in his car seat.

My crockpot of piping-hot spinach dip that had been lying on the back seat floor was not so lucky. Dip went flying and splattering everywhere, including all over

Andrew's car seat. Thankfully, he was still so tiny that I had placed his seat facing out the back window. Otherwise, the spinach dip would have burned his delicate skin instead of hitting the car seat.

The impact caused my body to go into a coma. An emergency room registered nurse (R.N.) named Bob happened to be standing in his friend's front yard and witnessed the whole accident. I asked Bob several years later if he had seen our cars collide. He told me he just saw my car land. Yikes! Apparently, the impact had launched my car airborne. No wonder it was scrunched!

Bob ran over to pull me out of the driver's seat. The teenager that had hit me was in a sport-utility vehicle. His car was crushed, too, but he was walking around. Bob saw green stuff all over the back seat of my car and thought the baby had thrown up, but it was just the flying spinach dip. He gave me cardio-pulmonary resuscitation (CPR) and made sure I was breathing. Then he waited for the ambulance to arrive. The ladies in the neighborhood passed Andrew around during the wait.

An emergency room nurse just happened to be standing there when I had my accident? Many would call that a coincidence or freak luck, but I call it a God-intervention. I told that story many times over the years when explaining the particulars of the accident. Why did it take so many years for me to see God's hand there? Was it my trauma or my lack of faith? Perhaps it was the way the story was relayed to me by Drew or my family, since I was not conscious to experience the trauma.

Before I moved from Louisville, my brother Dan was my primary-care physician. Apparently, I still had him listed in my wallet to call in case of emergency, so Dan got the call from the emergency medical services of Little Rock (E.M.S.) notifying him of my accident. My husband did not even know yet. Still, Dan was on the telephone giving E.M.S. my health and medical history. Drew only found out when he got to the party and Andrew and I were not there. He called our house and picked up a message from the hospital, saying that I was in the emergency room.

Within the next few hours, my entire family converged on Little Rock, hoping it was not the last time they would see their daughter/sister. The doctors said that if I made it through the night, I would probably survive. Some people have speculated that, as a runner, my excellent cardiovascular condition probably saved my life. Perhaps. I personally believe that God was not finished with me yet. He had a greater calling for my life than just to survive.

My accident was on May 10, 1997. I regained consciousness over the Fourth of July weekend. Coming out of the coma was a very gradual process. My first two weeks were spent in critical care on a ventilator. When I was able to breathe on my own, I was moved to a step-down unit with four other patients. My eyes were open most of the day, but in spite of appearances, no one was home.

What a journey the next few months would be! My dad tells me that while I was in the step-down unit, my legs jerked around wildly in my hospital bed. I told him perhaps I was dreaming I was running a race. I now know that is what happens when brain pathways are disconnected. My brain did not understand that lying down called for stillness.

The nurses did not want to strap me in my bed, so for my own safety, they put my mattress on the floor. That way I wouldn't have far to fall if my thrashing around brought me to the edge of the bed.

According to Dad, the first words out of my coma were not very gentle. The night nurse was checking my vital signs. I sat straight up in my bed and said, "Who the hell are you?" What a grand entrance into the world of conscious living!

My parents rented an apartment in Little Rock while I was in the hospital. They wanted to be able to accommodate family and friends when they flew down to see me. Mom stayed during the week, and Dad drove down every weekend, after his last patient left on Friday.

My parents said they rarely saw Drew at the hospital. I suppose he came at night after his work day was finished. I do remember him visiting one night with our baby, Andrew. In my memory, it was dark in the room, with light only from the hall. Just how late was it?

My first memory is of waking up in a bedroom with my mother sitting at my side in a chair, reading. I asked where I was. When she told me I was in a hospital, my first question was, "Where's Dad?" I figured that if it was a hospital, Dad could not be far away. No questions about Drew or Andrew. Did I even remember them at that point?

Once fully aware of my surroundings, I became keenly aware of my immobility. I did not even know how to use a walker yet. At first, I felt trapped in the bed. Then I discovered scooting on my bottom was an efficient way to move my body around. The social side of me wanted to know what was going on. So I would scoot out to the nurses' station and pull myself up to the counter. I had worked in hospitals for so many years; this seemed the logical place to find out what was happening. Then I would scoot down the hallway just for the exercise of it.

When I got tired, I would scoot back to my room. I always had the television on. Princess Diana had recently died in a terrible car accident. Her life was being remembered and her passing mourned all over the world. She was so young! That could easily have been me. At this point, I was so traumatized by my inability to walk that Princess Diana's death was just news on the television. This may also have been the first sign of my nearly all-consuming self-centeredness. Would I ever be able to be happy or sad for anyone else again, or were my physical limitations going to eat me alive?

Chapter 2

The Healing

Let us approach God's throne of grace with confidence, so that we may receive mercy and find grace to help us in our time of need.

Hebrews 4:16

I have divided this book into the three distinct segments that define each of us as human beings: BODY, MIND, and SPIRIT. In this chapter on my own personal healing, I will take a slightly different approach that was recommended to my friend by her licensed clinical counselor. This counselor saw being healthy as living within these four quadrants of our human nature: PHYSICAL, MENTAL, SPIRITUAL, and SOCIAL.

I will talk about my own personal healing within these four quadrants.

My Physical Healing...Sort Of

Recovery from a brain injury is different with each individual. Depending on what part of the brain is hurt, different consequences will occur. My brain injury is called a *contrecoup injury.* That means that the injury occurred in all parts of my brain. The majority of the damage happened in either the cerebellum, which controls my balance, or the brain stem, which controls my breathing and heart rate. I thank God for allowing me to retain my reasoning and intelligence.

From the day I got home from the hospital, I have been on a continuous mission to improve my mobility. My quest to walk normally quickly became an obsession. I talked in *The Light Through My Tunnel* of my crazy daily routine of going to the gym, along with an abundance of home exercises.

Once I moved back to Louisville, my daily working out continued. I was ashamed of how my body moved and worked continuously to improve it. I did physical therapy. I did yoga. I did an abundance of aerobic exercise and made sure I lifted weights at least twice, and preferably three times each week.

Then in 2010 I started my fitness business, Silver Strength®. Once, twice, and sometimes three times a day, I benefited from the strength and balance class I taught for my senior pupils. I always made sure I got my gym workout, though. See? I told you I am obsessed with exercise.

My muscles are strong and toned. Is my balance any better? Probably not a great deal, but I've learned to live with being unstable. The instability has become second-nature to me now. I have learned over the years how to catch myself when I'm ready to fall. I have learned numerous balance exercises, but have struggled to stick with them.

It's because a runner's mindset is ingrained in me. If my heart is not pumping harder, I don't feel like I'm really exercising. I lift weights and do calisthenics because I know they keep my muscles strong and flexible, but balance exercises are hard for me and remind me of what I no longer have.

That is no excuse! *"For the spirit God gave us does not make us timid, but gives us power, love and self-discipline." (2 Timothy 1:7)* Balance exercises are not going to change my body overnight. Just like praying, I need to fit them into my daily schedule. Surely I can squeeze balance exercises into my daily routine. Over time I will see the rewards for what I'm doing if I don't give up.

My Mental Healing

The healing of my brain has been an ongoing process. When I first came out of my coma, I had NO short-term memory. We still laugh about how my sister, Julie, had to reintroduce herself every time she re-entered my hospital room.

I knew the baby crawling around in the living room was my son Andrew, because family told me he was. It was several weeks before I actually remembered giving birth to him. That is something a mother just doesn't forget.

Other friends in Little Rock were so nice and gracious to me. It wasn't until I was looking through a photo album one evening that I realized I had known them before my accident. I thought they were all new friends! My short-term memory seemed to include anyone I'd met in the past two years, and that's the part of my memory that went missing for a while. My long-term friends I knew without question!

I still have trouble with my short-term memory today. Unless I call someone by name, over and over again, I cannot quickly recall it. My brain never stops trying to figure it out, though. Sometimes when I'm drifting off to sleep, the name I was trying to remember that morning will pop into my mind. Better late than never!

Memory wasn't the only mind issue I encountered. I felt damaged and different from everyone else. I still do, to some degree. The way I walk, my balance disability screams at people, making it very difficult to appear normal. People seem to like and even admire me, but with my poor balance and odd-sounding voice, it's hard for me to accept myself sometimes. I'm so very different from others. I always wanted to be special, but not THIS special.

After losing my relationship with my husband and son, I felt very abandoned. I felt that I no longer had any role in this life. My mental health score was at an all-time low when I lost my balance, my normal voice, my career, my home, my husband and my son. I should have seen a psychologist or therapist. Instead I turned to God to give me strength. I joined prayer groups and Bible studies, watched Christian movies, and read Christian books. I surely loved the Lord and was always overwhelmed with the kindness people routinely showed me.

I felt very isolated, though. I was not responsible for or to anyone or anything. That's a very lonely feeling.

Yes, I knew that my family and friends loved me, but we could go days, weeks, or even months without seeing each other. We all get caught up in our own routines. I certainly get caught up in mine. The only difference is that I come home at night to just me.

How could I involve other people in my world? While pondering this question, I innately kept doing what brought me enjoyment and a sense of control. I worked out at my health club five days a week. It gave me a daily routine and allowed me to be with other friendly gym-goers. I came home most days with a very positive outlook on life. I'll speak more about this later when describing my social awakening.

My Spiritual Healing

The most profound and cherished of all my improvements has been my spiritual healing. I have been a believer and part of the Christian Catholic church all my life. I said my prayers, went to church and tried to be kind to everyone. I led a very blessed life.

Nothing or no one had ever tested my faith. Enter brain injury, divorce and disability. Talk about testing! My life was changed in an instant. I could no longer do many of the things that had defined me. The family I had waited so long for was now gone. What did I have to wake up for every morning? What was my purpose for living? Why didn't God just take me home when I had my accident?

I believe with all my heart that God saved me with a purpose in mind. He's watching to see what I can do for him with this odd life he's given me. "Why do you want to help God?" you may ask. I gladly accepted all the blessings he brought into my life. Yes, he's thrown some real whoppers at me now. *"Shall we accept good from God, and not trouble?" Job 2:10 NIV*. Do I sound like the book of Job?

I have always thought of God like the earthly dad *EXTRAORDINAIRE*. Just like my earthly dad, I count on his guidance to keep me moving in the right direction. I realize that not all of us have a father we can look up to. God blessed me with a kind and wise man in my dad.

Was my disability some sort of discipline for something I'd done wrong? After pondering that for years, I don't think I was doing anything wrong. I think the Lord is trying to get me to do something good. He wants me to show others that you can indeed love your life when it's piled high with challenges. Just because I'm hurting doesn't mean I can't help someone else in pain. More importantly, I can show others that you don't necessarily have to walk with ease to be in the right place, doing the right thing.

God never promised us blue skies and smooth sailing. He promised us eternity with him after we've completed our testing time here on earth. Don't know what your test is? Think of what you struggle with. How can you make it better for someone else? How can you help those who are hurting? Do you ask for God's direction? We could all spend more time in prayer. I'm a big fan of the one minute anytime prayer. All day long, we can stop to give God thanks, ask for his mercy or seek his guidance.

My spiritual life was nothing exceptional until I was hit with so many life challenges. I see God's hand in the actions of my family, my friends, and even total strangers. I struggle with the simplest of things, like stepping off a curb. Others innately put out a hand or offer assistance. There's God! He's there in the embrace of friends, the sweet smile of a niece or nephew, the belly laugh with a friend at the gym.

What I said in *The Light Through My Tunnel* is still a reality. Even though I spend most evenings by myself, I never feel alone. Jesus is always just a breath or thought away. He is the one I want to impress; the one I want to appreciate me. I would be a lost and unhappy lady without God as the focus of my life. Of the four quadrants we try to satisfy in our life, the spiritual quadrant is the most life-sustaining for me.

My Social Side

I've always leaned toward being a loner in life. I never felt compelled to work out, shop, or even eat with anyone else. Growing up in a big family was fun and gave me constant companionship if I wanted it. From an early age, though, it inspired me to cherish my own privacy. I like being in my own head. My son Andrew says he has a daydreaming problem. Maybe he inherited it from me.

I'm not anti-social, though; I just prefer my own company. It's in my head that I usually get promptings from God, too. Now I feel like he's prompting me to be around others more. I get to interact with people all day at work and love it. I've lived by myself for over ten years now. I usually really like it. I have enough evening occasions out that I don't feel trapped in. I think I need a better balance of in … and out of my head, though.

My balance disability drives me inward to make sure that every step is secure. I've been known to walk right by people and not see or hear them. I become more outgoing when I'm sitting down and not concerned about my next step. Walking while talking can be dangerous for me, especially if I want to make eye contact with someone. That requires more balance than just looking forward.

That's the only legitimate excuse I have for being anti-social. Andrew tells me I'm sometimes unaware of what's going on around me. *Look around, Mary! Notice things!* I blame it on my selfishness. Nothing is more important than what I'm thinking about.

I've said many times that I never feel alone because I know that God is right there with me. Being with others, though, gives me the chance to spread his love around. I get new viewpoints on thoughts that are concerning me. I have the pleasure of making someone smile or laugh. I get to smile and laugh myself.

Like I said, I've always been a loner, but I love the feeling of getting in there and tackling something together. Time goes quickly when I'm enjoying someone else's viewpoint and humor. Most importantly, it gets me out of my head!

For several years after my accident and TBI, I was very reclusive. My family is quite boisterous, and I had become extremely soft-spoken and difficult to understand. So at family functions, I usually felt separated from the group. I was okay one-on-one, but it was difficult competing with a group. Eventually, I gave up and spent family time reading, watching TV, or exercising in the next room. Remember, exercising is my passion and obsession.

I quickly became more sociable when I started my fitness business, SilverStrength®, in 2010. I began leading exercise classes in senior homes and centers. Not only am I enjoying others' company, I'm on stage teaching a group of five to twenty residents. I get to do that two, or sometimes three times a day. I guess my reclusive days are over for now.

Being sociable again has made a most positive change in my outlook on life. We were all meant to live our lives with others, sharing and enjoying each others' gifts. My time with the men and ladies in my class causes me to think of the Bible verse we use at every Catholic Mass.

"May the grace of the Lord Jesus Christ, and the love of God, and the fellowship of the Holy Spirit be with you all." 2 Cor 13:14

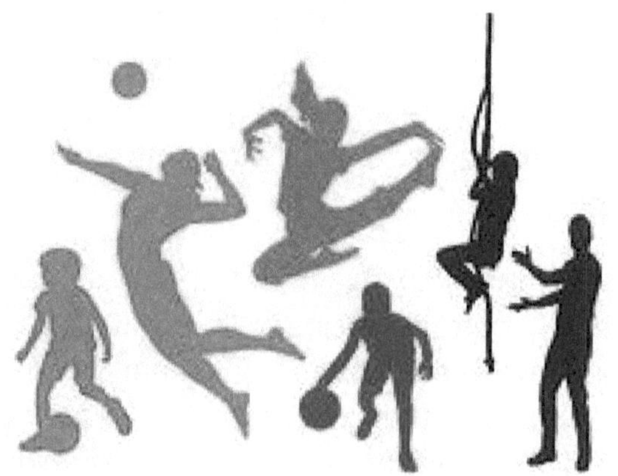

Chapter 3

Becoming a Healer

And we know that in all things God works for the
good of those who love him, and have been called
according to his purpose.
Romans 8:28

Parts of this chapter come directly from *The Light Through My Tunnel*. Why reinvent the wheel, right?

As a marathon runner and regular gym groupie, physical fitness was my life. I would show up late for social engagements in order to get my run in. All that changed when I suffered my traumatic brain injury in May 1997. I used to run an eight-minute mile. Now sometimes I can only keep my balance with a rolling metal cage called a walker. Otherwise I just walk extremely slowly.

I was upset and baffled. Why had this happened to me? I had so much! Life as I knew it … was over. I knew it was an accident, but it was so hard! I decided that this was not going to get the best of me.

God gave me a spirit of courage and determination. I was now in training for something bigger than a simple, little marathon.

Is this what my life had become? I did not work this hard training for distance races. Even though my balance disability kept me from running anymore, I discovered that equipment, like an elliptical or a treadmill with handles, could help me keep my aerobic fitness. Sit-ups, pushups and weightlifting required no balance, so I had no excuse for not doing them.

During all my years of recuperation, I remained a gym groupie. As I watched the personal trainers working with their clients, I knew I was as fit as they. I didn't have to walk to write a fitness plan, or demonstrate proper use of exercise equipment.

I longed for a way to help others again, even in my compromised physical state. I have read many books and articles about how to find God's will for your life. They all say to use what you are gifted in and what you are passionate about. I seem to be gifted to inspire others to try harder and my passion for physical fitness has long been established. This would be the perfect career for me!

I decided this would be my new purpose, and started studying for the personal training certification exam immediately.

My previous career as a pharmaceutical sales representative gave me an understanding of the body's anatomy and physiology, but memorizing new terms was very hard for me. My memory wasn't as good as I thought it was. Perhaps that was my brain injury, or perhaps my mind had become lazy from not studying for so many years. Whatever the reason, I had to take the exam twice before I passed the certification.

Today I am a certified personal trainer. My health club immediately put me on their payroll. However, if you cannot obtain the clients, you do not work. Who was going to choose me with a club full of able-bodied trainers? My marketing background went right out the window.

How do you promote a trainer with a balance and voice impairment? All that training

and studying! Had I done the wrong thing? How could I promote myself? Seems the Lord had a different plan for me. His plan surfaced only after I stopped telling Him all the reasons why it would not work out.

I am personally comforted and challenged when I read Moses speaking in Exodus 4:10. *Moses said to the Lord, "Pardon your servant, Lord. I have never been eloquent, neither in the past nor since you have spoken to your servant. I am slow of speech and tongue."* I knew God didn't need perfect speaking ability to help me touch the lives of others.

I truly believed that God had put this dream in my heart. How would he make it a reality? A woman from the Vocational Rehabilitation office suggested I teach group exercise classes in senior homes. Voc Rehab even bought me a portable sound system with a microphone. The microphone helped the seniors to hear my soft voice over the *oldies* music.

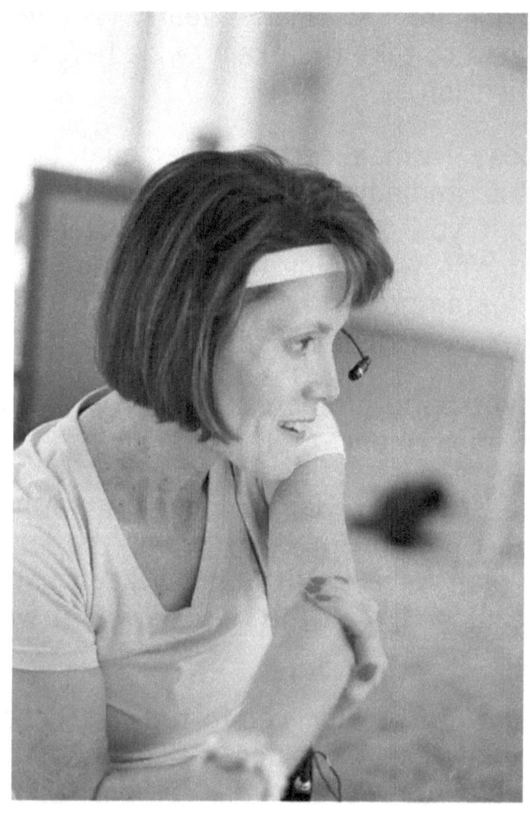

Regular exercise is very important for older adults. The old saying is true: *"If you don't use it, you lose it."* I seem to inspire the seniors in my class. They figure if I can do it, they can at least try. In the process of leading my classes, I'm getting a balance workout myself.

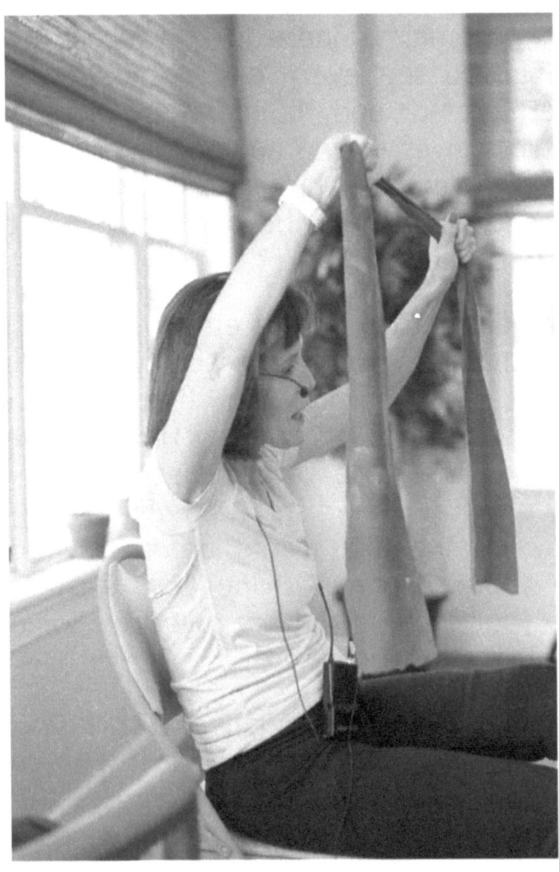

Over time, I was able to add more classes. I started out teaching muscle toning and flexibility. Then I added more and more balance exercises. Balance work is so important for older people. And for me too! The exercises I teach help me as much as they do my students. My years as a physical therapy patient gave me lots and lots of cues to use when I teach my classes.

A personal trainer—on a walker? It is not something you see every day. While my students aren't athletes or body builders any more, working with seniors gives me an audience that appreciates what I have overcome through regular exercise. I am able to encourage them beyond what they thought they were capable of.

My disabilities do not embarrass me or make me feel ashamed when I am teaching. They have led me to a new purpose in life; inspiring and encouraging those I serve. Many times I have heard myself using the same verbal cues with my classes that my physical therapists used while trying to get my body moving like it did before my accident. *Elevate your rib cage. Bring your hips forward. Squeeze your shoulder blades together.* Sometimes I sounded like a broken record.

God tells us in Romans 12:21 , *Do not be overcome by evil, but overcome evil with good.* My new purpose as a *wounded healer* uses the issues I've struggled with to motivate and encourage the seniors in my class. By showing them the exercises I've done to regain my mobility and strength, I have shown them ways to maintain their own.

To continue living independently, these seniors need to keep their bodies moving on a regular basis, just like I do. I help them keep their bodies in the proper alignment to make the tasks of everyday living easier. If caught slouching in my class, they are sure to hear me say, *Elevate your ribcage* for the 15th time.

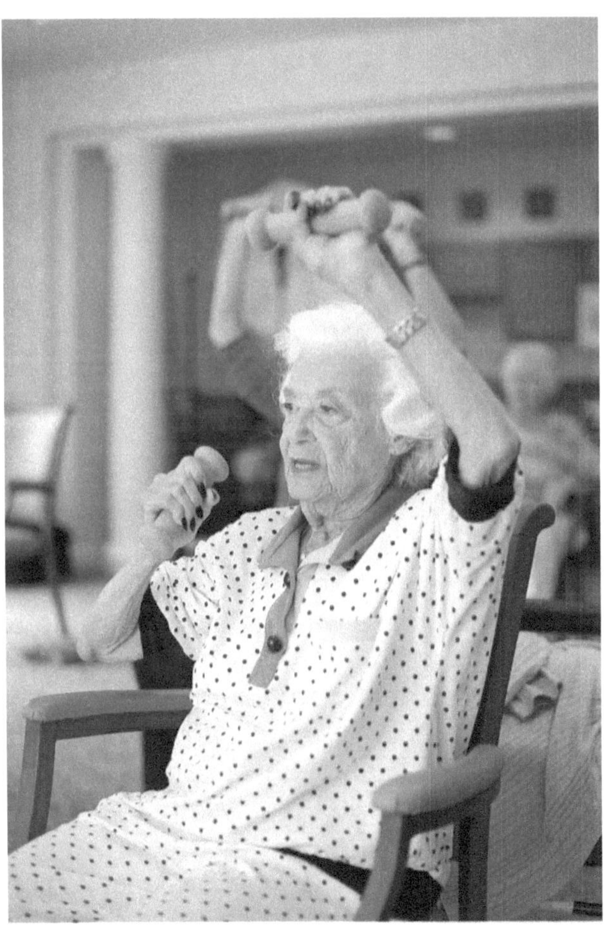

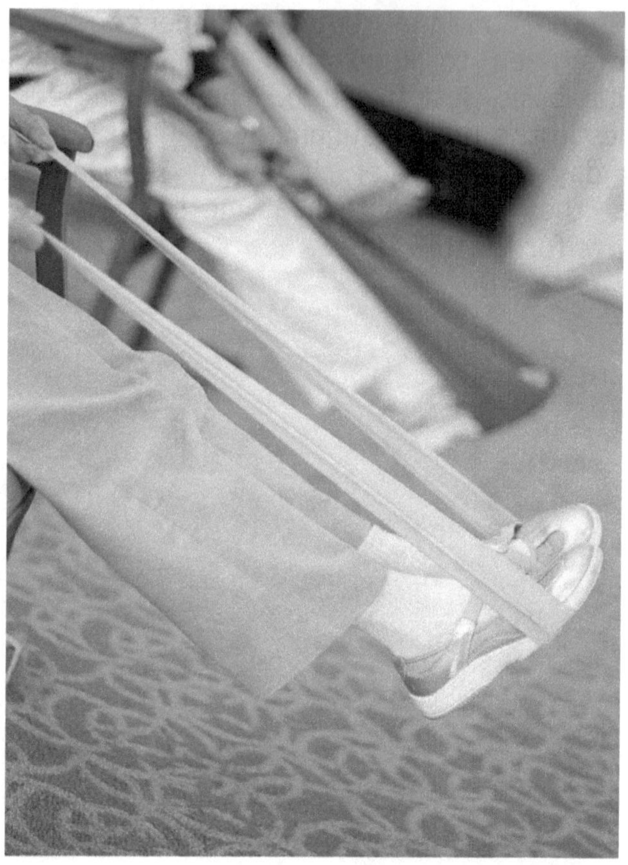

Occasionally, a senior in one of my classes will let me know they are walking better or able to climb stairs since starting my classes. It seems to give them confidence that they can have mastery of their body moves through practice and proper execution of the move. As I lead the classes, I am practicing the proper body moves for myself, too. I get a free physical therapy session every time I teach a class! My body moves have become more and more fluid and my balance is better since I began teaching. My body is exhausted by the end of the work day, though. Holding myself in good posture for several hours still does not feel natural.

Improved muscle tone and flexibility are not the only benefits of taking my classes. It is also a great opportunity for them to build camaraderie with the other residents. We share fashion tips, food recommendations and current events, all the while commiserating about why we have to exercise. We laugh, joke, and truly enjoy each others' company. I wake up excited to see them every day. Teaching these seniors has really enriched my life!

I looked forward to going to work every day. Since May 10, 1997, (my accident) I have relied on people's assistance to get around in life. I still do, to some degree. What a boost it is to my confidence to have others watching my moves to help them get around more gracefully.

The majority of my pupils have better mobility than I do, yet they rely on my instruction for the proper execution of moving their joints and muscles. One day a newspaper photographer was filming my class. I got nervous and lost my balance. I sat down immediately, as did my entire class. I still laugh thinking about it. They sure do follow their instructor's every move!

I have found my new purpose in leading these classes for seniors. I show them how to remain strong and flexible. They show me a wonderful outlet for helping people again. These ladies and men have become like a second family to me. I seek their advice on things. They watch out for me. My days of being a long-distance runner were taken away to make room for a new and more meaningful purpose. My race time is slower now, but much more rewarding.

About a year after I had started my senior fitness business, SilverStrength®, my dad remarked that when people survive a trauma like mine, they usually count their blessings, find peace with it and make the best of what they have left. *"But not Mary! She's going to make a career out of it."* That's how I became an afflicted healer. In the next chapter, I will describe others who have used their personal challenges in life to bring healing to others.

Chapter 4

There Are Others

*For we are God's handiwork, created in Christ Jesus
to do good works, which God prepared in advance for us to
do.*

Ephesians 2:10

I explained in the previous chapter how I became an Afflicted Healer when I was able to help my senior students improve their fitness level and ability to move. I was able to do this despite my own physical challenges with an imbalanced body.

The world has many afflicted healers. You may know one yourself. These are the individuals who use their talents or abilities to help others to reach their full potential, despite challenges they personally endure. I have had the honor of knowing some of these healers personally. The first afflicted healer I will mention, I do not know personally, but he has been a source of inspiration and hope for my life since I came upon his website on the Internet a few years ago.

Nick Vujicic

Nick Vujicic is an Australian–born Christian evangelist and motivational speaker. He was born with tetra-amelia syndrome, a rare condition that left him with no arms or legs. He is one of only seven people worldwide who live with this condition. Nick did have two feet that enabled him to grab things, turn pages, and do various other functions. As he got older, he was able to operate an electric wheelchair, computer and cell phone with his foot.

I can only imagine the teasing and bullying he received growing up. With the love and support of his parents, Nick had a reasonably normal childhood … the only *normal* he had ever known. When he was seventeen years old, Nick's mother gave him an article she'd read about a severely disabled man and how he managed his life. Not long after, he began speaking at his prayer group. That was only the beginning of Nick's journey that would inspire and bring hope and change to others.

Nick has an international non-profit organization called *Life Without Limbs.* Through this mission, he brings the message of the saving and healing power of Jesus Christ to people all over the world. I have one of his mantras taped on the mirror in my bathroom that says, "If God will not show me the miracle, He's going to make me the miracle for someone else." Nick also has a secular motivational speaking company named *Attitude is Altitude.*

Life was not always rosy for Nick. He questioned whether God even had a purpose for his life. He suffered with depression, extreme loneliness and actually attempted suicide once when he was younger. I myself am very happy and relieved that he is still here today to give me a renewed outlook on this precious gift called life.

Growing up in Christian homes, Nick and I are very similar in our devotion to a life lived for Jesus Christ. As I mentioned, I don't know Nick Vujicic personally. I feel a bond with him, though, as we have both found our purpose and our comfort in Christ. I am humbled and astounded at all that Nick has done for the Lord in his life. I was blessed to have thirty-seven years of normalcy before my disability. I have family, friends and a wonderful son to share parts of the journey with me. Now Nick has inspired me to do more to bring God into the lives of the people I meet. Perhaps this book is one of those tools.

When researching Nick Vujicic on the Internet, I noticed that he was born in 1982. I was born in 1959. That means I'm old enough to be his mother. One normally thinks of a mother as giving both practical and inspirational advice. People are always telling me I am an inspiration, but Nick, young enough to be my son, has inspired me to embrace his positive, Christ-like outlook on life. Nick inspires me to "be the miracle."

Dr. Kimberly Alumbaugh

I've been blessed to know personally the rest of the afflicted healers I will describe. My next description is of my own sister-in-law, Dr. Kim Alumbaugh. I'd like to say that our family has the afflicted healer gene, but Kim is married to my big brother, Dr. Dan Varga. There is no blood relation. There is however a spirit of making the best of what life hands you, by using those circumstances to help others.

Kim was born and raised in the small town of Higginsville, Missouri, 40 minutes from the metropolis of Kansas City. She grew up happy and loved by her parents, sister and two brothers. Content as she was, Kim always felt there was a big, wide world out there calling to her. So after high school, she left Higginsville for the University of Missouri. After graduating, she went on to their medical school for four more years.

Then it was time to choose a medical specialty. Kim felt she was getting the best of both worlds when she chose Obstetrics/Gynecology as her specialty. She would have the challenge of practicing and perfecting surgical techniques while still being intricately involved in patient care and education. Best of all, she would play a primary role in bringing new life into the world.

While completing her residency at the University of Louisville, Kim met and fell in love with my brother, Dan. I can still remember the party bus we took to transport all of the Louisvillians over to Higginsville for the wedding. It was the chance for Kim to showcase the hometown that made her the person she had become.

After their marriage, Kim and Dan immediately began trying to fulfill their dream of having a family to share their love with. She knew from her medical background, that it might not happen immediately. It did not.

After consulting fertility specialists, she ultimately discovered that her body had gone through an early menopause and that she no longer produced the eggs necessary to begin a new life. Kim and Dan were devastated! They refused to believe that their dream of bringing children into the world was shattered. Of course, there was adoption, but Kim was a young, healthy woman completely capable of carrying and delivering a healthy child.

After much thought and prayer, they decided to try *in vitro* fertilization. They would take another woman's eggs and combine them with Dan's sperm to make a fertilized egg to then be placed in Kim's uterus for developing into their child. The *in vitro* process produced three viable fertilized eggs. When implanted into Kim, the first implementation resulted in a miscarriage. The second implant resulted in her cherished twins, Sam and Noelle. They were perfectly healthy and adorable. Dan and Kim wondered if they should just accept this gift from God and not try any more.

In the meantime, Kim threw herself into her OB/Gynecology practice. She was now an expert in women's healthcare. She loved working with her patients on ways to become healthier and took her role as a surgeon very seriously, making her patients feel very secure in her abilities. I remember Kim operating on me for a routine gynecological issue. After administering the sedative in the operating room, my last memory was of Kim holding my hand, telling me everything was going to be fine. Then I woke up in the recovery room.

After much more thought and prayer, Kim and Dan decided to try implanting the final fertilized egg into her womb. That implementation resulted in yet another healthy, smart, and adorable child they named Tess ... Theresa Marie. They were inspired to use the name Theresa because my aunt Nancy had prayed a novena to St. Theresa asking for a healthy baby for her and Dan.

Kim has delivered over 3,000 babies, including all of her nieces and nephews. My son, Andrew, was the exception, since we were living in Little Rock, Arkansas. Because of her own fertility issue, Kim has a keen interest in women's reproductive health. She has truly become an afflicted healer serving all the healthcare needs of the female patients she serves.

Dr. Alumbaugh is also one of the 'experts' that will contribute her knowledge on women's health later in the book.

I didn't have to look far for the rest of the afflicted healers. Every year I have the honor of selecting another brain-injury survivor to receive the Mary Varga Award. The recipient of my award is a brain-injury survivor who has used their gifts and talents to help others in some way. Each of the following individuals received my award in a different year. They were not just giving assistance to others, but actually helping specifically those who are also afflicted.

Alex Nauert

Alex is a staff sergeant in the United States Marine Corps. He is currently on reserve status, but Alex is the epitome of an afflicted healer when on active duty.

Several years ago, Alex's life changed forever during a routine mission to bring back a damaged tank. He was riding in a tank when it struck an improvised explosive device, an IED. Alex was riding at the top of the vehicle and remembers nothing of the event other than a white flash of light. The next thing he remembers was being in a hospital twenty minutes later.

He could barely talk or see, and he felt as if his back had snapped in two. He had suffered a traumatic brain injury (TBI). Thankfully, he only required hospitalization for seven days, but he spent several more weeks in rehabilitation. He declined the Marine Corps's offer to send him home and chose to finish out his deployment in Afghanistan.

He felt driven to give back for all the help and reassurance the Marine Corps had given him when he was injured in the line of duty. He not only received the Purple Heart but also the support and encouragement of the entire Marine Corps.

He wanted to reach out and advocate for other injured Marines to give them the same compassion he had experienced as a wounded warrior, so he became part of the Wounded Warriors Initiative.

In Germany, Alex acted as the first contact for Marines injured in the line of duty. He was their champion/liaison through their initial recovery. Once, he met the plane transporting a double amputee who was so seriously injured he was not expected to live to see his family again. Miraculously, the injured Marine defied all medical expectations and was taken off a ventilator within a few days. Alex and a fellow liaison would sit with him to telephone his family. He could not speak yet, so Alex would hold the receiver to his ear so he could hear his family's voices. The injured Marine would respond by squeezing his fingers. Alex then became the voice of the wounded Marine by speaking his words to the family. He described the scene as being extremely moving.

Alex wants to use his experiences as a wounded warrior and give back to the Marine Corps for their commitment and support of him during his struggles. A military life remains his dream, and he has indeed found a job where he can assist other wounded warriors with the same exemplary care and support he received when he was injured in Afghanistan. As he puts it, "I'm just returning the favor!"

Ginette Allen and Kasey Hamsley

I group these two afflicted healers together because their affliction, a traumatic brain injury (TBI), led them both to a career in occupational therapy. Both Ginette and Kasey suffered their TBIs because of car accidents. Ginette was riding in a car when it was struck by another. Kasey was playing around with friends and fell off the hood of the car, on her head.

Ginette's Recovery

Two weeks after being admitted to the hospital, she was transferred to Cardinal Hill Rehabilitation's Brain Injury Unit. This ended up being her home for the next 5 weeks. She had to learn how to live again. With left-sided weakness due to the brain injury and a right shoulder injury, this proved to be very challenging. Of course, the brain injury also left her with little-to-no short-term memory and poor safety-awareness, which made the road to recovery even more daunting. Fortunately, she had dedicated therapists and a supportive family, which had a significant impact on her outcomes.

After returning home from her initial hospitalization, Ginette's journey continued with outpatient occupational and speech therapy. She can remember the moment that she asked her OT what it would take to become an occupational therapist. Ginette decided that this terrible accident did not happen in vain. She wanted to use the experience to help other people who had survived. She recalled her dismay when an OT at Cardinal Hill told her she "knew how it felt" to be frustrated by the rigors of therapy. Ginette knew that she could use the same phrase with a brain injury survivor and really know how it felt! Ginette went to college and graduated as an occupational therapist 5 years later!

Throughout her career, Ginette has had many opportunities to share her story with patients and their families, hopefully impacting them in a positive way. At the end of the day, she could not imagine another life for herself and she looks forward to seeing how she can continue to impact the world around her, especially through being a mother to her children and her job as a pediatric occupational therapist.

Kasey's Recovery

Kasey had to be stat-flighted to the University of Louisville for an emergency craniotomy. She had to wear a helmet for several months to protect her damaged skull. During that time, Kasey also had two strokes. After spending eight weeks in ICU she had to relearn how to move, walk and talk.

Kasey's occupational therapist worked with her daily to show her sometimes new and different ways to manage the activities of daily living. Taking a shower; using the bathroom; dressing; styling her hair; putting on make-up, all fell under the occupational therapist job description.

Both Ginette and Kasey chose occupational therapy as a career after being the recipient of the care and service given to them as patients. Both have had the chance to work with other brain-injury survivors and feel a close camaraderie with all patients who are dealing with the same challenges that they did. They are able to share their recovery to give hope to patients who can't see the light at the end of the tunnel.

As an occupational therapy assistant, Kasey tries to pass on to her patients the words of Winston Churchill: "Never, never, never give up."

Paige Raque

The final afflicted healer I will mention is actually a healer-in-training. Paige is also a brain-injury survivor who received my award at the annual Brain Ball.

Paige was a student and varsity cheerleader for Penn State University when she suffered her brain injury during her sophomore year of college, after falling out of a fifth-floor window.

In October of 2012, she spent about two weeks in critical care in Pennsylvania before being transferred to a rehab hospital when she emerged from her coma. Ultimately, Paige was transferred back to Frazier hospital in Louisville, finally being discharged just before Christmas that year. She immediately began the outpatient day program with the Frazier NeuroRehab Program.

A traumatic brain injury was not the only injury Paige sustained in her fall. She also broke her pelvis, her sacrum, and a few ribs. She fractured her tibia and had small fractures in a few vertebrae. Realizing how lucky she was not to have been hurt much worse, Paige responded with *"God is good!"*

Paige spent much time with her therapists and relied on their every word for a complete recovery. Since she was still undecided on her career choice, her therapists encouraged her to follow an academic path to become qualified as a therapist. At this point Paige knew without a doubt that she wanted a career that allowed her to help others. She also knew she wanted something in the medical field.

Now the question became what type of therapy she would choose in order to make the biggest impact in helping patients. Paige had developed strong relationships with each speech therapist that helped her along her journey. She continues to be inspired by the impact they had on not only her recovery but the role they continue to play in her life today.

Paige completed her Master's degree in Speech Pathology in May 2018. She currently works at Cedar Lake with adults with intellectual and physical disabilities, and loves it! Always seeking to do God's will in her life, Paige summarizes, "I thought God was going to open the door for me to work with people who had sustained a brain injury because this was my personal experience and I felt passionate about giving back to this population. However, as he so often does, God had other plans! I truly know that this is the door God has opened for me. I love all of the individuals that I work with and feel blessed to use the knowledge and skills I have been given to help them. I feel I am making a difference and giving back in the place that God has chosen."

Chapter 5

BODY, MIND, SPIRIT

The remainder of *The Afflicted Healer* is divided into Body, Mind, and Spirit. To live life to its fullest, we need a healthy balance between all three components. Only when the segments are working together can we achieve the peaceful and active life of purpose for which we all strive.

I will first address the BODY, the most visible area for afflictions or challenges to present themselves. Sometimes others may see what we're struggling with, but oftentimes not. My hope is that this portion of the book will highlight different strategies for getting and keeping your body moving the way it was designed to travel. I have asked physicians, therapists and personal trainers to share the methods and strategies they use with their own clients or patients.

In my first book, I referred to Baptist Milestone as my home away from home. My physical fitness and mobility have evolved in the ten-plus years that I have been a member there. Sometimes I seek their professional guidance; most times I go about my own fitness routine. As you read through the chapters in this book, you will find information that may raise questions in your mind. The staff at any health club is trained and able to respond to your questions.

The personal trainers at Baptist Milestone are certified through the American College of Sports Medicine (ACSM). In their publication, *ACSM's Exercise Management for Persons with Chronic Diseases & Disabilities* (fourth edition 2016), their goal is to help physicians use exercise, as easily as they prescribe medication, to assist in overcoming chronic conditions.

Since exercise prescription is not covered by a majority of health insurances, my book will help by outlining many forms of exercise that will help improve the lives of those dealing with chronic conditions. Please review with your doctor or healthcare provider before beginning any exercise program.

Have some fun with this! For exercise to become a part of your daily life, you must enjoy it...and the friends you will make along the way.

Chapter 6

What's Your Doctor Telling You?

For wisdom is more precious than rubies, and nothing you desire can compare with her.

Proverbs 8:11

What are your doctor's orders? We place our very health in their hands, but do we truly follow their guidance and direction?

Meet three physicians practicing in Louisville, Kentucky, as they give direction on the importance of making regular exercise a part of your total plan for health and wellness.

Dr. Stuart Urbach

Internal Medicine

Dr. Urbach has been my neighbor since I was a little girl. His family lived just up the street from mine. I had the privilege of working with him professionally when I was a pharmaceutical sales representative 20 years later. Then we ended up living in the same condominium complex ten years ago, after he and his wife Sherri sold their home.

The condominium complex was built just blocks from my childhood neighborhood. It was my first experience with home ownership since I had my brain injury and had moved back from Little Rock, Arkansas. How nice it is now to be living right next door to my former neighbor!

Now read what Dr. Urbach tells us about how vital exercise is in maintaining an active life. He should know! He's been at it personally for over 90 years.

Stuart Urbach, M.D. FACP

I am Stuart Urbach, a physician specializing in Internal Medicine. After a 38-year stint in private practice I joined the U of L Med School full time faculty for 15 years, and for the last 10 years have been doing odd internal-medicine jobs at the Metro Jail, at the Louisville VA Hospital, and in a practice that treats opioid addiction. I also do some teaching of undergraduates in the Med School.

Mary asked me to write about the changes I have seen during my long medical career in the way medical professionals view the role of exercise in maintaining good health.

First, let us discuss hospital care: Hospitals report their size by the number of beds within their walls. Certainly bed rest is a part of the care of our sickest patients. But as the patient improves with treatment, bed rest that was appropriate at the beginning may no longer be needed. Sometimes inertia takes over and we may be slow to get eligible patients out of their beds.

Eleven years ago, at age 82, I was injured in a bike/auto accident. I was banged up a bit, but nothing too serious. Because my helmet was broken I was admitted to the hospital for a possible head injury. I was placed on total bed rest with wires attached to my chest and limbs. I did nothing active for three days, and when discharged I had great weakness and difficulty just trying to walk around the block.

Unneeded bed rest with lack of exercise is a health hazard, especially for the elderly. As little as three days of bed rest with no exercise can cause weakness, muscle shrinkage, increased risk of clots in veins, decreased ability of the heart to keep blood flowing up into the brain upon standing, increased risk of falls, confusion and dementia.

Many of our sickest patients can be helped to a chair, can sit up to eat or watch TV, or be helped to a bedside commode. They can be taught bed exercises to use even when on total bed rest; and they can use an overhead trapeze bar to help with turning. In a recent scientific study a group of frail hospital patients wore monitors that counted their steps. The patients who walked 900 steps or more per day did not suffer any increase in their frailty, while those who walked less than

900 steps per day declined. (900 steps could be walked in about eight to twelve minutes).

Many years ago we would keep patients on bed rest longer than it was needed. Some women were at rest for two weeks after a delivery, and heart attack patients rested as much as five weeks. Paul Dudley White, cardiologist for President Eisenhower, helped to change habits and to establish "early ambulation" as a standard for good medical care.

Bed rest is "bad rest" when it is not needed. Being up and about and getting appropriate exercise is therapeutic.

Dr. P.K. Cherian

Cardiology

I met Dr. Cherian at a book signing for my first book, *The Light Through My Tunnel*. He explained that he was buying the book for his wife, since he did not take the time for any pleasure reading. A few weeks later, he reintroduced himself and told me that his wife gave the read book back to him, urging him to read it himself. I was honored that she liked my story that much.

Several months later, I asked Dr. Cherian's personal trainer, Alison, if she would be interested in being a guest author for a new book I was considering. I wanted to write a book that spoke to individuals with all kinds of afflictions, showing them how to maintain an active life with purpose. I think Alison was as excited about the idea as I was.

Alison told me that Dr. Cherian offered to be a guest author for my book as well, speaking from a cardiologist's perspective. I was thrilled! I still don't think that Dr. Cherian (I call him P.K. now) has read my first book. Perhaps he will read *The Afflicted Healer* since he is now one of the guest authors.

Dr. P.K. Cherian
Norton Heart Specialists

Recommendations for Physical Exercise.

Physical activity is a key component in achieving a healthy lifestyle and disease prevention. One in four don't exercise; rich nations fare the worst. This puts them at greater risk for diseases like heart disease, hypertension and diabetes. Also, there is decline in mental health and quality of life for people who don't exercise enough. Heart disease is a prevalent disorder, but also a preventable disorder. Guidelines recommend participating in some type of muscle-strengthening activity at least twice a week, along with moderate aerobic exercise for 150 minutes a week and 75 minutes a week of vigorous working out. Exercise and healthy diet can lower the risk of health problems such as diabetes or cardiovascular disease, including more than 40 of the most common chronic health conditions encountered in a primary practice. This can add more than 10 years to life. It has been shown that risk of heart disease is highest in individuals with low cardiopulmonary fitness when compared with traditional risk factors such as hypertension, diabetes, dyslipidemia, etc. Each MET (Metabolic Equivalent of Tasks) increase (3.5ml/kg/min) in cardiorespiratory fitness can reduce cardiovascular and all causes of mortality by 8 to 17 percent.

A MET (Metabolic Equivalent of Tasks) expresses the energy cost of an activity, and therefore the intensity of that action. It indicates the amount of oxygen the muscles need to perform that activity.

Here we will focus more on an exercise program for people with health issues. At a regular doctor visit, the healthcare provider only has a brief window of time for physical activity counseling, not more than 20-30 seconds. However, a healthcare professional can ask pertinent questions to prescribe the right dosage of physical activity to patients for prevention and treatment of the disease process. For people with chronic health conditions, he/she can provide them with specialized guidance on how to safely exercise with a given condition. The healthcare provider should be the example and influence his/her patients by participation in exercise as well.

To assess the (PA) physical activity levels, simple and rapid tools are available. I can assess the physical activity level of the patient in less than one minute. This consists of two simple questions: "On average, how many days a week do you engage in moderate to strenuous exercise like a brisk walk, and on an average how many minutes do you engage in exercise at that level?" These two screening questions will provide the healthcare professional snapshot information. It will determine whether the patient can or will be meeting the current PA guidelines of 150 minutes each week.

Exercise is beneficial in treating dozens of diseases such as diabetes, hypertension, obesity, heart disease, Parkinson's disease, multiple sclerosis, etc. Even though one may have a medical condition, the healthcare provider can determine the current physical activity status of an individual and then the desired intensity of physical activity. Most individuals now need no further screening if they wish to participate in low-to-moderate intensity activity. However, greater attention may need to be given to high-risk individuals who wish to engage in vigorous physical activities.

Determining the Individual's readiness to change:
#1: Patient has no intention to be physically active. Promote being more physically active by discussing the health benefits, emphasizing pros and cons of changing their behavior and helping work through the cons of being physically more active.
#2: Patient is thinking about becoming physically active, is ready to listen to a healthcare professional or a trainer.

#3: Patient is active and making small changes, but not meeting PA guidelines. A trainer in the gym will be very effective.

#4: Patient is meeting the PA guidelines, but has been for less than 6 months. Strengthen their ability to change and ability to fight urges to slip back.

#5: Maintenance. Your guidance in linking them to community resources and more specifically to exercise professionals is a key strategy. Fitness goals should be adapted to individual situations.

Starting the Program:

Walking is the preferred initial form of exercise because it requires no special training or special equipment. To start, a target heart rate of 20 beats above the resting heart rate for 30 minutes is adequate. The FITT-VP principle (Frequency, Intensity, Time, Type, Volume, Progression) is utilized to benefit the participant. Frequency and time will be considered as 5 days a week for 30-60 minutes of moderate intensity exercise or 3 days a week of 30-60 minutes of vigorous intensity. If you can walk and talk it is moderate intensity. If you can walk and talk breathlessly, it is high intensity.

Choose a low-impact type activity such as walking, cycling, or water exercises. Start with short sessions of 10-15 minutes and gradually build up to 20-40 minutes, 3 or 4 days a week. Take as many breaks as you need.

Stop exercising if you feel chest pains or angina and contact a physician. New research shows patients with moderate obstruction to left ventricular outflow tract (HOCM), compensated heart failure can exercise under supervision after evaluation by a physician.

Resistance Exercise Programs:
Frequency: 2-3 days a week.
Intensity: 1-3 sets of 8-15 repetitions for each muscle group.
Modality: 5-15 lbs free weight or equivalent or few lbs by machines.

There are programs available in the community. One could contact health clubs and fitness facilities, YMCA and local community centers.

Do not hesitate to ask the personal trainer questions:
Do they hold a 4 year degree from a university in exercise science?
How long they have been a personal trainer?
Are they certified in first aid and CPR?
Do they have liability insurance?

Have a nice workout!!

P.K. Cherian MD, FACC
Board-certified cardiologist with Norton Cardiology
Practicing cardiology for nearly 40 years

References:
Kirk Evans, MS

Clinical Exercise Physiologist, Certified Strength and Conditioning Specialist

16 years working in cardiac and pulmonary rehabilitation

Braunwald's Heart Disease

Hurst's The Heart

Topol's Comprehensive Cardiovascular Medicine

Exercise in Medicine

Swain, DP et al. Comparison of Cardioprotective benefits of vigorous versus moderate intensity aerobic exercise.

Wolters et al. ACSM's Guidelines for Exercise Testing and Prescription.

Dr. Darryl Kaelin

Physical Medicine and Rehabilitation

As a brain injury survivor, Dr. Kaelin's specialty in Physical Medicine and Rehabilitation is where I began my recovery in Little Rock, Arkansas, twenty years ago. Even though obstinate and out of touch at the time, I still liked and trusted my physicians. My focus and short-term memory were oftentimes out to lunch during the early days of my recovery.

Dr. Kaelin's advice is both practical and sometimes inspirational for me twenty years out. Would I have listened at the time of my trauma? Probably not. I was so immersed in what I had lost and finding the quickest way to get it back. My only interest was in fixing it.

I suppose that's why God gave us caregivers. Sometimes a caregiver is also a memory-keeper.

Now read what Dr. Kaelin suggests for living a purposeful life when the life you had has suddenly changed.

Darryl Kaelin, M.D.

Physical Medicine and Rehabilitation

As a physical medicine and rehabilitation physician working with patients who have experienced significant changes in their function, I am often faced with the question, "Why do bad things happen to good people?" Experiencing a catastrophic injury or illness can turn your life upside down. Frequently a person will go from being completely independent and productive in their life to being completely dependent on others for their self-care and mobility.

When a person's thinking, behavior, strength, and mobility changes it creates a sudden challenge to one's self-identity. They hear others say that they aren't like they used to be. They begin to ask "Who am I now?" This kind of loss results in the grieving process. In medicine, we think of this as going through the stages of denial, anger, bargaining, depression and finally acceptance.

As a physician working with patients that experience this sudden and oftentimes lifelong change it is important to recognize patients going through the grieving process and help them to understand it as they go along that journey. Often these individuals will come to some acceptance that although they want to continue to get better and lead more productive lives, they can be happy with the person they are, even if it is different than the person they used to be. Medical care, rehabilitation, healthy lifestyle, and counseling can lead a person to acceptance and toward a more satisfying life. Acceptance usually occurs when a person finds meaning in the illness or injury they have suffered and creates a new purpose in their life going forward. In other words, there could be a reason this bad thing occurred.

In keeping with the theme of this book, I remind all patients that it is important for them to resume and maintain balance in their life. This balance lies between their physical, intellectual, emotional, and spiritual makeup. The rhythm and balance in life is what makes us happy.

Physically there are medicines that help a person to think more clearly and recover faster. There are also medications that are needed to prevent complications such as blood clots or future strokes and heart disease. It is important to work closely with your primary care physician and your specialist in order to understand the purpose behind each medication. This increases your confidence and likelihood of being compliant and taking the medicines as directed.

Just as important, and more important in some cases, exercise is medicine. There are numerous studies that show how exercise will not only improve your physical, mental and emotional well-being, but works better than many medicines to reduce future complications and hospitalization.

Very often a person living with chronic illness or disability will need direction in the safest and most appropriate way to exercise given their condition. The American Heart Association recommends that all adults get approximately 30 minutes of aerobic exercise per day five days per week (150 minutes/week). This is relatively easy for some people and very hard for others. Remember, anything you do is better than nothing.

Your 30 minutes each day can be broken into 10- to 15-minute intervals 2 to 3 times daily. Walking is generally the best exercise. If you can walk at a pace where you are huffing and puffing but can still talk to someone walking with you, that is best. If not, any walking will do. If walking is too difficult I often recommend a recumbent bicycle (see picture). The seat makes balancing easier and provides good aerobic exercise.

If your legs are impaired or you can't afford a recumbent bike, then consider an arm ergometer (see picture). This doesn't work quite as well, but does give you some aerobic activity.

One of the best places to exercise is in a swimming pool. This can be either outdoor or indoor. People with heart conditions, seizure disorders, and significant balance problems should consult their physician before attempting water exercise. Swimming is not necessary and a trainer or physical therapist can show you what exercises to do standing up in a pool. It is best and safest to do this type of exercise with a partner. There are many group water exercise classes in the community.

In order to see improvements one must vary their training program and always try to exercise harder and faster over time. Exercising the same way at the same pace over time doesn't usually work. Don't let anyone tell you that you won't get better after one or two years. I have seen many brain injury and stroke survivors make significant improvements many years out from their onset when they begin to change up their exercise program.

When your thinking and talking have been affected by illness or injury, cognitive and language therapy provided by a speech pathologist can be very helpful. Accepting cognitive and behavioral deficits requires a great deal of humility, but receiving treatment can generate tremendous improvements. Rehabilitation for problems that affect the brain and nervous system takes months and even years to reach maximum benefit. Don't give up. Exercising your brain regularly is as important as exercise is to your body. Reading, playing games, and even computer and video games can improve your attention, memory, and visual skills.

Chronic disability resulting from illness or injury often results in social isolation. Your roles in your family, among friends and at work all change. People around you become uncomfortable with how to act or what to say to you. This is especially true for teenagers and young adults. Life seems to be passing you by while you are stuck at home. This often leads to emotional problems such as depression and anxiety. When these issues start to interfere with your daily life and relationships, medicines may be necessary, and can be very helpful. Counseling with a psychologist can also be valuable, but nothing works better than the two together. Be willing to talk to others. Seeing a perspective other than your own and getting feedback is very important in coming to acceptance.

At the onset of disability and during the grieving process people are often focused on themselves. "Why did this happen to me?" "Will I ever be able to walk again?" "When will I get better?" "Can I go back to driving/work?" Finding meaning in your disability and setting a new purpose in life focused on someone or something outside of yourself often improves one's mood. I encourage people to get out of the house and socialize. Don't be ashamed or afraid to talk about your illness or injury. This makes other people feel more comfortable in asking questions and understanding what you've been through. Friends, family, and neighbors often want to reach out and reconnect, but don't know how. By reaching out first you often open the door for them to come in. It is only through relationships with people and God that we are truly happy.

As physicians we have a unique opportunity to use our medical practice as a ministry. Medicine is a science and an art. Too often we focus only on the science. Doctors are not trained much about the spiritual side of people, but we can use our own faith and experiences to guide and direct our patients as they struggle on their spiritual journey. Physicians should believe in holistic care, and this certainly includes spiritual well-being as well as physical, mental and emotional. Because not everyone's belief systems are the same, physicians must try to meet their patients where they are. It is important not to be judgmental. I often ask my patients about their faith and encourage them to spend time praying, meditating, or just connecting with God and nature. In our busy, chaotic world, spending some quiet time contemplating life and praying can be extremely valuable in finding meaning and helping reset the course for the future.

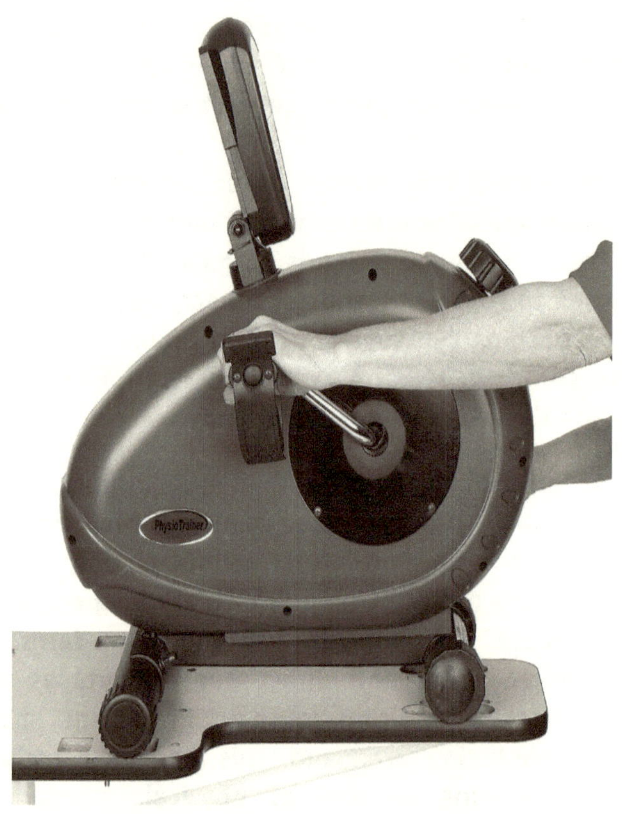

Arm ergometer

Recumbent bicycle

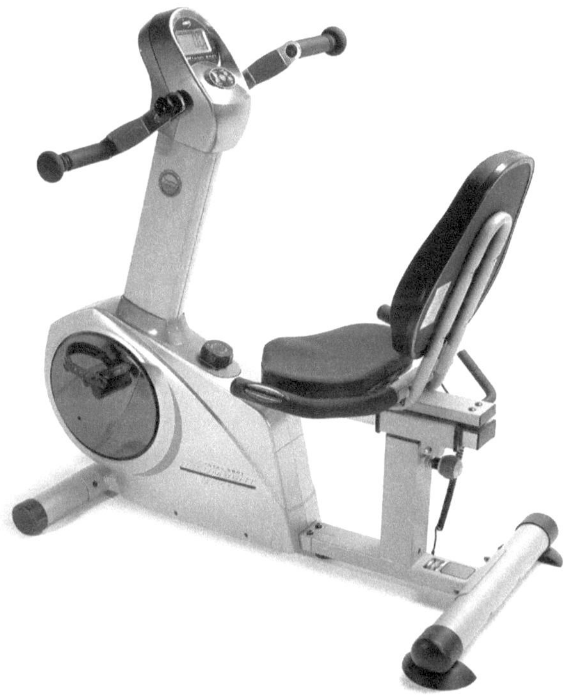

I can
accomplish
anything

Chapter 7

Embracing Womanhood at Every Stage

*Jesus turned and saw her. "Take heart, daughter,"
he said, "your faith has healed you." And the woman was
healed at that moment.*

Matthew 8:22

Another physician I asked to contribute to my book is Dr. Kim Alumbaugh. Kim is also my sister-in-law, married to my older brother, Dr. Dan Varga. Kim was my personal physician in Obstetrics/Gynecology when I moved back to Louisville after my brain injury. I was blessed to have her as my doctor for just over ten years before she moved with her family to Dallas, Texas.

The Afflicted Healer is divided into three separate sections comprising BODY, MIND and SPIRIT. In the pages that follow, Kim also defines a woman's self as being the compilation of her body, mind and spirit. She gives several examples of how women neglect their own bodies in attempting to be all things to all people.

Read on to learn what we often do and how to then avoid undermining our own precious female health.

Dr. Kim Alumbaugh

Obstetrics and Gynecology

When Mary asked me to write this chapter, I admit, I was unsure how to proceed!

After 25 years of woman-care, which lessons of the thousands learned offered the greatest opportunity for retelling? I sensed that the spirit of my message needed to be an empowering one. I finally decided to explore, from a female perspective, the integration of our bodies, our minds, and our spirits.

Through 25 years of rendering care, I found that most infirmities were underpinned by misgivings and insecurities. Some weeks more referrals were made to psychological counselors, exercise physiologists, sexual therapists and nutritionists than were made for ultrasound, mammogram or outpatient surgery! Daily, the close connection between the patient's physical condition and her mental satisfaction and spiritual well-being was revealed. Directly connected to many of her physical life experiences was a variable commitment to her "self" and to her comfort in her universal role womanhood.

The examples for this connection were often presented by what they did not say. Their maladies often revealed where they had been cheating themselves, and where they had been replacing what was missing from their lives and their childhoods with ineffective solutions that were causing them physical pain. The complexities of their lives became evident when they began to talk. When their chief complaint read "none, just annual exam" it was sometimes as if the entire exam was a just a preamble to the real problem. Having given them their instructions for the upcoming year, with my hand on the doorknob, and searching for anything I had overlooked, I sometimes felt like there was still an unasked question. . This sensation would make me return to the rolling stool in front of them, with an invitation to "Talk to me, what's going on?" It was then that I was the best doctor I could be, because I had detected something unsaid, yet necessary for their healing. I am often reminded that taking care of oneself is truly hard work! Time is a luxury we women rarely afford ourselves. So, STOP! Make a list of all the things you have to do. RIGHT NOW! EVERY 'TO DO' on your mind. DON'T TURN THE PAGE. DO IT NOW AND ORDER IT BY PRIORITY! PLEASE!

Now, hand someone the list. Have them read it back to you. As a women's health practitioner, I will bet that among the 'to dos' on your list, your personal physical care items rank nowhere near the top. In my experience, women only truly take care of their own health concerns once everyone else's needs and desires are taken care of and everything else on their endless 'to do list' is done. No new mother seeks to remove exercise from her life! She allows it to slip away through responsibility. Her need to support and nurture her new family becomes paramount. She often only goes to work or participates in outside activities because of the referred benefit to her family. She endures painful job conditions, unsatisfied educational desires, abusive personal situations and physical malady caused often by inattention to her health solely, and mistakenly, to perform in her role as the ultimate nurturer.

We allow the real responsibilities and false obligations of our lives to lead us from our own paths and we daily celebrate and are celebrated for the fact that we "die to try!" We daily witness friends whose professional lives increasingly demand more and more of them through travel, added responsibility, and leadership positions. So great are these demands that our friends do not exercise nor seek the annual health care they deserve. The women in our lives allow their self-care to slip away because they see it as a self-indulgence far less important than the responsibilities they assume they have been given. We quite frequently lie to ourselves that "Once our job concerns are met we will indulge our selfish desires for self-care." Second of the "notes to selves," ladies: self-care isn't selfish, and our job concerns will never fully be met!

Neither the dutiful wife who makes sure that dinner is on the table and the house is perfectly tidied following her 9 to 5 existence, nor her husband coming into his perfectly maintained castle should be at all surprised when her selfless efforts result in a complete abnegation of her sexuality and libido. Where in the world would she find the energy to first overcome the residual body dissatisfaction created by her self-inattention, and further, when would she have time to muster up a bit more flame in the bedroom in the face of homework, bedtime, and bath time? Any husband's surprise that this previously raging fire has died should understand it often has more to do with the depletion of the wife's fuel source than with her missing desire. If vacation returns the flames, then that crazy life you are leading is surely what is putting them out!

Every day we women create a mantra of delayed gratification assuring us that we are being good mothers, good workers, good wives, good daughters, good caretakers, good public servants, and good church participants. The list of entities we must satisfy before addressing our personal needs simply does not end. Add to this delayed gratification, the perverse belief that our own needs are somehow selfish and unloving, and you can easily see why our perennial garden regrows more weeds than flowers, more work than respite, more pain than pleasure! We need to understand that our false sense of selfishness and obligatory self-denial is depriving our children, those we mentor, and our friends, all of whom are looking to us for guidance and mentorship, of an example of a life worth emulating.

We refuse to recognize our worth. The cure is as simple as remembering that if the tree or root should die, it cannot then bear fruit! What in our minds seems selfless is in fact far more selfish, because it deprives our bodies of what we need to walk on our own paths. It deprives those we love of our guidance and our good example. We need to stress the importance of self-care to all of those we love. Our life's good example teaches them how to be. Instead of allowing ourselves to be drawn into progressively disabling relationships through misguided selflessness, we must learn to protect our own vitality so we do not prevent them from seeing our best selves.

The concept of caring for ourselves is really a simple matter. It involves avoiding ignorance, addressing our universality, and acknowledging change. The practice of our self-care is quite another thing. Ladies, we cannot just talk these concepts, we have to walk them!

Avoiding ignorance is different from seeking knowledge. Medicine is a constantly changing field. It is difficult to stay abreast of current care, but that is your physician's role. The magazines may say one thing, the news media may blare another, and quite often your doctor's practice may depend on her experience. Unfortunately, her desire to bring you up-to-date often depends on the busyness of her day and the number of complaints you present.

With each visit, remember to write down your concerns. Face to face with your doctor you will probably forget everything you wished to ask! If your doctor does not offer advice on how to be your best healthy you, then you should ask them for that advice! Woman care is not just about addressing your problems, it is about helping you manage the difficulties we all know are coming! Each yearly exam should include an update of your past history to inform your doctor's future decision-making. Although you may believe that your physical exam is the reason you have come through the door, information from the actual physical exam is almost useless without the integration of your symptoms and problems! Turning your office visit into a guessing game based on your physical exam is not helpful. Speak up before your exam and offer what is on your mind! If you do not agree with the doctor's reassurances, be prepared to explain why you believe your case seems different. A bell will then go off in your physician's mind and it will lead her to retrieve even more important information about a potentially adverse condition. How will the doctor know if you do not speak up? Trust me, the mind reading class has been removed from every medical school curriculum! Third of the "notes to selves," ladies: your physicians are not psychic.

A good doctor will always look further than a physical exam. They know each woman's physical is unique to them and reflects a woman's past and current stage of life. Year-to-year changes are subtle, and they are best noted by the person who daily experiences them. Usually, they do not indicate an abnormal condition, but they do invite your doctor to consider the usual life cycle changes experienced when these physical signs occur. For example, examination of the vulva of a mature woman following childbearing often shows a relaxation of the area under the urethra. A woman cannot usually feel this specific change, although she might sense something is different 'down there.' The presence of this change may or may not be symptomatic. However, it never ceases to surprise me how one simple question at the time of the physical exam "Do you leak urine when you cough or laugh?" is often met with the answer, "Of course, I have for years!" Immediately I return to the chart to check why I have ignored this poor suffering woman's listed complaints, only to find she had never once offered it as a problem! I am often overcome by guilt for my inattention and failure to probe, and respond "How could I have let you live with something we could have easily fixed?" This remark is usually met with, "Dr. Alumbaugh, I thought everyone had this after they had a kid, or after they went through menopause!" Although part of this is a result of the insurance requirement to separate problem visits from annual visits, I advise that during your annual exam you speak up about your problems and if needed return to get them fixed. Believe me, you are worth it.

Caring for ourselves challenges each of us to accept our life cycles and acknowledge the experiences we will have sooner or later. Good doctors give us a heads up, but we often fail to recognize that the most important source for the majority of that information is the other women in our lives.

However, even with them, we let our embarrassment impede us. The very personal nature of a condition occurring in our 'private parts,' the same private parts held by all women, prevents our forthright questioning and certainly impedes learning new information from one another that would enlighten us. Shouldn't we as women make the concept of our 'private parts' a bit more of a universal experience? We women miss an extraordinary opportunity to support each other when dealing with periods, having better sex lives, having difficulty conceiving, preventing unplanned pregnancy, being afraid of childbirth, learning to breastfeed, dealing with changes to our vaginas, vulvas and breasts, dealing with changes in our emotions and our stressors, and dealing with menopause and the subsequent remarkable life that lasts for thirty years beyond menopause! Sharing our amassed knowledge we become stronger and our knowledge becomes more refined and true. Our shared experiences could help us help each other, if only we replaced our fear of inappropriate sharing with the concept of inappropriate withholding.

There are so many conditions a woman does not have to endure! Most can be easily overcome with lifestyle modification, medication, in-office or outpatient surgical intervention. When women avoid sharing information because of their uncertainty they limit their opportunities to receive good health care. The acceptance of the outdated adage "some things you just have to live with" is a missed opportunity for healing. The gender ignorance we subject ourselves to out of fear, embarrassment, and insecurity can be changed by sharing with each other, and our physicians. The good ones in both groups will hear you and those who don't can be replaced!

Early on we should recognize that there is a difference in acknowledging our basic female nature and accepting its dysfunction. Pain is not our gender-driven cost of being alive! Menstrual cycles, pregnancy, breastfeeding and menopause are beautifully complex and unique and are expected life events for a woman. Painful periods, bleeding with clots, recurrent pregnancy loss, horrible PMS, no cycles for months on end, painful intercourse, vaginal dryness, leaking urine on one's self, chronic constipation, lack of sexual drive and lack of sexual satisfaction, pelvic floor relaxation, inability to lose weight, depression, chronic fatigue, and many others are not expected requirements to be fulfilled simply because we are women!

Any expression of our oneness is both reassuring and empowering. One of the best gifts any mature woman can give to a newly menstruating frightened teenager, or a terrified mom-to-be, is a sense of our shared experience, a sense of what is normal, and the empowerment to speak up and out on what is confusing and painful. By acknowledging the togetherness of our mutual paths, no matter the difference in our experiences, we begin to testify that being a woman is truly a blessing.

Chapter 8

Get Moving

*May the God who gives **endurance** and encouragement give you the same attitude of mind toward each other that Christ Jesus had.*

Romans 15:5

As an adolescent, I would jump rope on our screened-in back porch in the afternoon before dinner. I would jump over and over again. Just five more minutes! Just five more minutes! Little did I know that I was setting the stage for the daily endorphin rush I would experience years later when I became a runner.

I didn't take to running as naturally as I did jumping. I asked my brother Dan how I could get myself to run further than half a mile without losing my wind. He ran cross-country for St.Xavier High School. Surely he could tell me. Dan figured the best way to show me was by doing it.

Before we started our run, he told me to stay on his heel. He was running so slowly that I kept trying to pass him. *"Stay on my heel!"* he would scream. "I want you to run so slowly that you're embarrassed when cars pass you." So I made myself go slowly. When we finished our jaunt, he told me we had just completed a mile and a half. That was a mile more than I had ever run.

I kept running at a slow pace. I ran further and further. I never got winded, and after a few minutes, the endorphins (adrenaline) would kick in. Then I felt like I could run forever! Eventually, my gait and speed naturally got faster. I always started slowly, though.

The first race I ever ran was a two-mile track in Seneca Park. I was so nervous I almost turned back on my drive to the starting line. I continued, though, as I was meeting my friend Nelson for the race. It was so much fun to be out there huffing and puffing with a hundred other runners, and I conquered my fear of racing. Then I started racing 5 Ks, 10 Ks, half-marathons and ultimately marathons. I knew I wasn't going to win, so I made myself, as always, start slowly, for the first quarter-mile anyway.

This is the same principle I follow with any cardiovascular exercise. My balance won't allow me to run or even walk briskly anymore. I do start slowly on the elliptical machine, the treadmill, or the stationary bike, though. Then if I want, I can pick up the pace after a few minutes; then slow down again at the end of my time.

I no longer train for races. My goal is to keep my heart strong and my weight down. That usually means about 20-30 minutes of cardio each day. That is my self-prescribed cardio program. Now let's hear what Alison Cardoza, ACSM-Certified Personal Trainer, has to say about cardiovascular fitness.

Alison Cardoza, ACSM Certified Personal Trainer

Jump rope, running and walking are some forms of exercise that get our heart pumping! Cardiovascular endurance is the ability of the heart and lungs to supply oxygen-rich blood to the working muscle tissues, and the ability of the muscles to use oxygen to produce energy for movement. Walking on the treadmill or marching in place are examples of low-intensity cardio exercise that increase heart rate and burn calories. If you are doing cardio exercise to burn calories, one pound is equal to 3,500 calories. So to lose one pound a week, a daily treadmill workout must burn off 500 calories each day. For beginners, start by walking around your neighborhood or on a treadmill. Ten to fifteen minutes would be best at first and work up gradually to avoid injuries.The next day, evaluate your body and increase the minutes to challenge your cardiovascular system. For the best benefit, and for a more intermediate to advanced workout, walk, jog or run at a moderate pace for 30 to 60 minutes every day of the week.

Cardiovascular exercise reduces the risk of conditions including obesity, high blood pressure, and type 2 diabetes.

Aerobic and anaerobic are the two forms of cardiovascular exercise. Aerobic exercise is intended to improve the efficiency of the body's cardiovascular system in absorbing and transporting oxygen. Examples of aerobic exercises are running, swimming, dancing, kickboxing, hiking and cross-country skiing.

Anaerobic exercise consists of brief intense bursts of physical activity, such as sprints or weight lifting. It is fueled by energy stored in your muscles through a process called glycolysis.

There are 3 basic energy systems of the body.

1. ATP-CP (phosphagen, which is an immediate source). This system supports brief, high intensity activities such as sprinting. This is an anaerobic activity.

2. The Glycolytic System provides energy for activities that are longer in duration and lower in intensity, like strength training. This is anaerobic activity.

3. The Oxidative System supports long-duration, lower-intensity activities like walking or long distance running. This is aerobic activity.

The three systems work together to ensure there is a continuous and sufficient supply of energy for all our daily activities.

Elevating your heart rate by doing cardio exercise causes endorphins to be released, which reduces stress and improves your overall heart health.

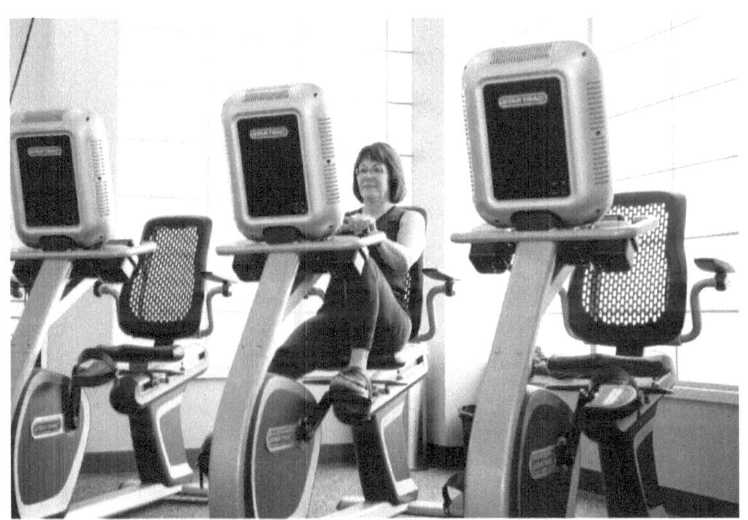

Indoor Biking

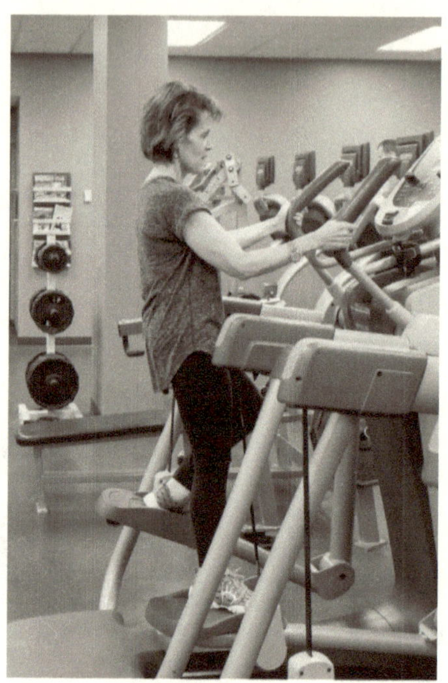

Elliptical

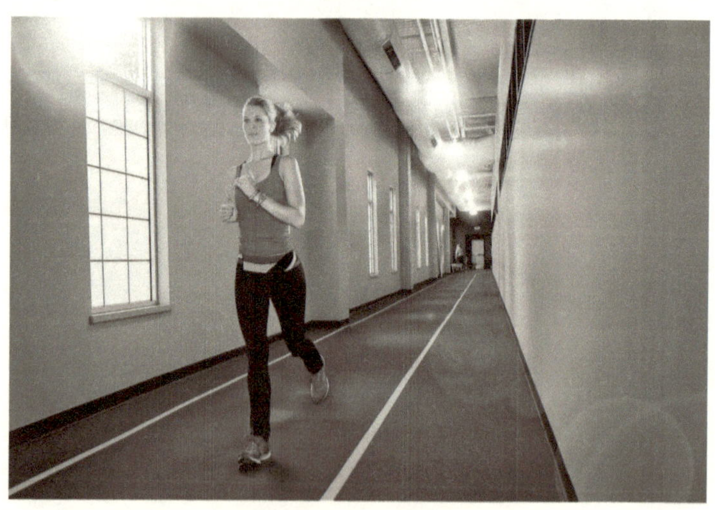

Indoor Running

Chapter 9

Get Strong

Those who hope in the Lord will renew their strength. They will soar on wings like eagles; they will run and not grow weary, they will walk and not be faint.

Isaiah 40:31

Strength Training

I have been following a strength program since I was in my early thirties, but had been running for ten years before that. What persuaded me to begin lifting weights? Being strong has never been a concern of mine. Being THIN was, however. Once I discovered that muscle burns more calories than fat, I was all in!

As a runner, I evaluated every fitness program based on the number of calories I would burn. I guess you could call me an *aerobic junkie.* Weight lifting is not an aerobic activity like walking or running, but it does set the stage for your body to burn energy more efficiently. If you continue to do it regularly, muscles become more defined. So now you're not only stronger, you look stronger, too.

I recommend starting a strength training program with the guidance of a personal trainer. They can show you proper form in weight lifting. I cringe every time I see another weight-lifter doing repetitions quickly in an effort to get them done. To gain any muscle strength, you must move the weight slowly when exerting force AND when relaxing. That's how to tone those muscles up!

Now read what Alison Cardoza, ACSM-Certified Personal Trainer recommends for getting your muscles stronger.

Alison Cardoza, ACSM Certified Personal Trainer

Let's admit we all have stood in front of a mirror and flexed our bicep muscle. For some of us, this motivates us to want to head to the gym and get more muscle in our biceps. For others, we may feel proud of our progress and are pleased to see what reflects in the mirror.

As a personal trainer, I ask my clients what they feel is the perfect body. Many say "thin" and "muscular." Every single body is different. I inform my clients that there is no such thing as the perfect body. If they are fueling their body with healthy nutrients, getting around eight hours of sleep a night, drinking water daily and avoiding unhealthy choices, then they are being the best version of themselves. "Thin" or "muscular" does not

necessarily define healthy. Staying active and eating healthy foods will help you be the healthiest version of yourself.

Did you know that when you work your muscles, you actually create little tiny tears in your muscle fiber? Rebuilding and challenging your muscles responsibly makes them stronger. I know some of you may be thinking, OUCH! No way do I want to tear my muscles! As long as you listen to your body and gradually increase weight, your body will heal and this process actually makes you stronger. The more you tear, the more you build muscle. This can leave you feeling a little achy and sore. Completely normal! Resting and applying heat to the muscles soothes the pain. Also, fueling your body with protein after a workout helps build your muscles.

Every strength training program is different for each person. When working with clients that have specific needs, I evaluate and design a program specifically for the individual.

Three types of weight training programs

There are three types of strength training programs that I recommend for you to strengthen your muscles. Choose the one you are most comfortable with and to which you feel you can commit the time required. With all strength training programs, the amount of weight is different for every individual. The correct amount of weight for a standard weight program would be a weight you can handle for three sets of 8-12 repetitions having difficulty ONLY with the last few repetitions in the last set. Begin with a weight light enough to keep proper form for numerous repetitions. This will take some trial and error to find the correct weight.

The first type of program I am going to introduce is high weight/low repetitions. The amount of weight is determined by the amount of reps you can do 8 to 10 times. This program focuses on white fast-twitch muscle fibers, meaning your body is building more muscle. An example of people who have a lot of white fast-twitch muscle fiber are Olympic sprinters and crossfit athletes. A crossfit athlete is someone who performs various functional movements at high intensity. Examples of crossfit workouts are movements that reflect the best aspects of weightlifting, running, gymnastics and rowing.

The second strength training exercise would be for endurance. This caters to individuals who want to be leaner and tend to do activities such as long distance running, cycling or swimming. The repetition range will be a weight that you can do 22 to 25 times for three sets. Again, use trial and error to come up with the correct weight amount. It will be lighter than you expect. Remember you'll be performing a high number of repetitions for three consecutive sets. This training modality focuses on red slow-twitch muscle fibers, which use oxygen to produce energy for muscle contraction.

The third and final weight training program focuses on movements that are explosive and powerful. The red slow-twitch and red fast-twitch muscle fibers are involved, and help the body produce a lot of energy! With a rep range of 12 to 15, the weight should be challenging toward the end of the third set. These are people that are lean but still muscular. Many people aspire to be lean and defined. This type of training will help you achieve just that!

Before starting any exercise program, consult your doctor. You do not have to work with a personal trainer; however, if you are just starting a training program for the first time, I would advise you to meet with a trainer to ensure proper form. The two most popular options for strength training are machines and free weights. The advantage to machines is that they are exercises you can generally do by yourself and it's easier to establish a circuit of exercises. The advantage of free weights, although initially more difficult to have proper form, is that you activate more of the small stabilizer muscles next to major muscle groups.

Strengthening these small stabilizer muscles is important to prevent injuries, maintain balance and is generally done after injuries during the rehabilitation process. Strength training improves posture, bone density, and muscle mass as well as releasing endorphins and improving overall health and well-being.

In the gym, always warm up for 5 minutes before beginning your strength training program. Walking, marching in place or riding a stationary bike warms up your muscles, helping to prevent muscle soreness or injury. It is important to do the warm up for only five minutes so your body does not get fatigued before you begin.

Be sure to work different muscle groups each day. Muscle groups need at least a day of rest in between workouts. Machines such as Chest Press, Lat Pull-down, Row and Leg Press work multiple large muscle groups. When working large muscle groups, do not do more than three exercises per major muscle group per day. Feel free to change those 3 exercises as frequently as you would like. Free weight exercises such as dumbbell bicep curls, triceps kickback and calf raises, work smaller muscle groups. When doing these exercises, breathe and exhale on the exertion. Be slow and controlled, 2 to 4 seconds on the upward motion and 2 to 4 seconds on the downward motion.

I design programs for my clients that cannot always make it into the gym. They may have osteoporosis, hypertension, and other health obstacles preventing them from being able to leave their home every day. If you cannot make it into the gym, here are a few exercises you can substitute at home with similar results.

1. Arm circles are an exercise to help strengthen the deltoid muscle, biceps and triceps. Arms are in a T position. Circle clockwise one minute and reverse.

2. Wall sit is another strength training exercise you can do at home. You want to start out with 10 seconds and work your way up daily. Keep good form. Knees should be in line with ankles, back should be glued against the wall. Make sure you are breathing in through the nose and out through your mouth!

3. Wrist strengthening exercises are important. If you do not have access to barbells, cans of soup can be a substitute. Keep elbows glued to your side. Place your palm in supination position (palm faces up to ceiling). Flex the wrist 15 times. Next, flip your wrist over and do one set of 15 extension wrist exercises in prone position.

4. Walking while holding onto dumbbells

5. Bent and straight leg raises with a dumbbell resting on upper thigh

6. Hold onto lightweight dumbbell and punch down your hallway and back

PIC: These strength training exercises elevate heart rate gradually and give your body a great workout.

Stay hydrated with water before, during and after your workout.

Overall, a strength training program should be designed specifically for the individual. It improves balance, stability, bone mass, and increases metabolism, burning fat off the body. By stressing your bones, strength training can increase bone density and reduce the risk of osteoporosis. Incorporate strength training into your schedule to improve your overall health and well being! Flex those muscles in the mirror and feel proud of your hard work!

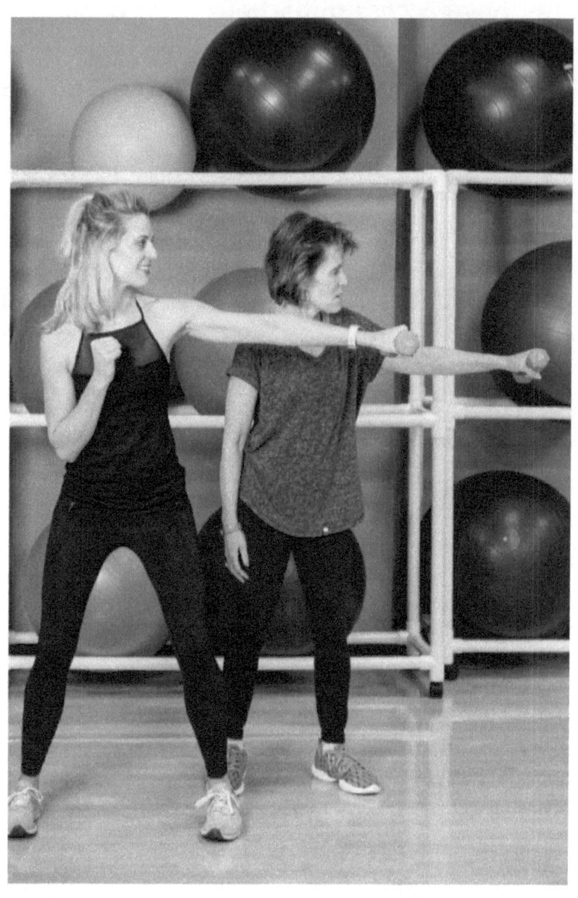

Punch/Side Steps with weights

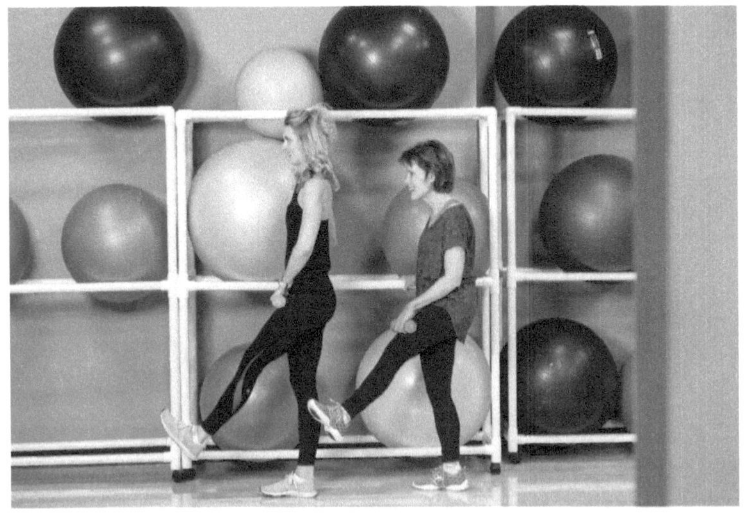

Weighted straight leg lifts

Everydayaffirmations.org

I can
succeed

Chapter 10

Getting Fluid

As a runner, I always did a quickie hamstring and calf stretch. If I was feeling conscientious, I would stretch my quadriceps as well. If I had 50 minutes, I spent 48 minutes running and two minutes stretching. I was young (30ish), flexible and not overly concerned with getting a proper stretch.

That all changed when I turned 50. Was it getting older or maybe the fact that I can no longer move around as quickly as I used to? Whatever the reason, now my leg muscles seem to scream at me to stretch them. So now it is a regular part of my daily workout.

My education to become a Certified Personal Trainer also taught me that lower back pain or soreness is often times caused by tight hamstring muscles. Just one more reason to make sure to get a good leg stretch.

Now let's read what flexibility tips Alison Cardoza, ACSM-Certified Personal Trainer has to share.

Warming up and stretching before and after a workout are essential. Your body requires stretching prior to an activity; do so in an active warm-up such as marching in place. Stretching before exercise prevents injury, while stretching afterward increases flexibility. Your body must be warm and loose before an activity to prevent injury.

After a workout it is beneficial to do slow, static stretching. Stretching helps release stress, tension and lactic acid in your muscles and prevents muscle soreness. It is important to hold your stretches for at least 30 seconds. You should not bounce when you are stretching. Each stretch should be static, holding still. Inhale and exhale slowly to oxygenate the muscles and prevent delayed-onset muscle soreness, which can occur a few days after a workout. These are some of my favorite stretches to do after a workout.

1. Calf Stretch—"Push the wall away stretch"

Visualize that you are trying to "push the wall away."

Arms are straight, both hands are on the wall. Take a few steps back and dig the right heel down to the ground. The left knee is in front, bent. Visualize the right heel squishing a marshmallow to the floor, slowly digging the heel down, releasing tension in the gastrocnemius, the calf muscle.

After 30 seconds, switch legs.

2. Hamstring Stretch—"Hike your leg Up"

Place your leg up on a stair in a stairwell. Keep the leg straight. The goal is to have the leg hip level. If the standing leg appears to bend, the leg being worked is up too high. Lower and stretch. Work your way up to a higher level as you progress.

This stretch can also be performed in the supine position, lying face up.

One leg is straight on the exercise mat and the other is vertical. Keep the leg straight, glute on mat. Extend leg toward your body and stretch hamstring muscle.

This exercise can be performed with a personal trainer or done solo. If you are on your own, a rope around the foot helps stabilize the leg and helps you get the maximum result.

If a trainer performs this, he or she can gradually increase the range of motion with PNF stretching (Proprioceptive Neuromuscular Facilitation). This helps improve the muscle or tendon's elasticity, flexibility and range of motion.

3. Tricep stretch—"Across the body"

Stand and gently, without tugging, place one arm across chest and gently stretch the triceps muscle.

Hold 30 seconds, inhaling through the nose and exhaling through the mouth.

4. Quadriceps stretch

Place right hand on left foot, bend knee and pull foot upward to stretch quadricep.

5. Stress release and shoulder roll.

Roll your shoulders forward 5 times and reverse 5 times. Shrug your shoulders up and down 5 times. This helps release tension in the neck and shoulders.

Stretching daily will improve your life. Change your life with cardio, strength training and stretching daily!

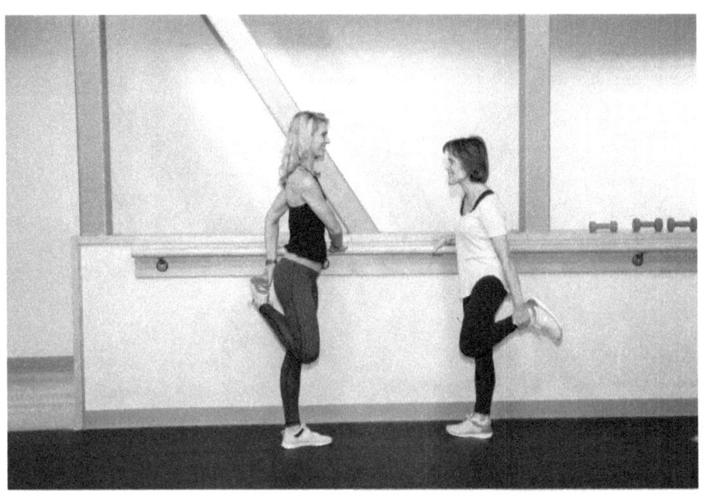

Quadricep Stretch

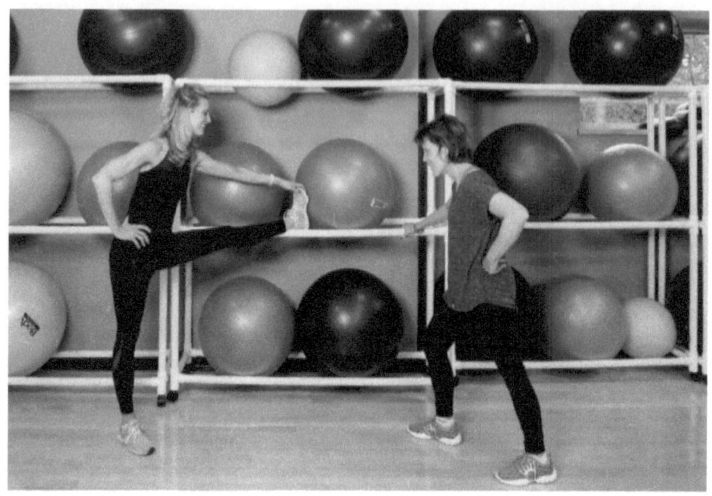

Hamstring and calf stretches

Chapter 11

Keeping a Balanced Body

Honest scales and balances belong to the Lord; all the weights in the bag are of his making.

Proverbs 16:11

Walking on the grass; walking in snow; stepping down off a curb. These are some of the things I have not been able to do without assistance for over 20 years. Like most people, I did not appreciate balance until I no longer had it. It was only then that I learned that the cerebellum of our brain controls our balance. Apparently that's one of the parts I damaged.

Balance is a product of three sensory functions working together. The vestibular system, which is located in the inner ear, detects rotational movement of the head and provides the body with information related to spatial orientation. The visual system has the obvious job of allowing us to see where we are standing, moving, etc., in relation to the world around us. And proprioception allows the body to have a sense of where it is in space, even without looking. Proprioceptors include both motor and sensory nerves. Thus, proprioception can be improved through regular exercise, specifically balance training.

My goal here is to show you ways to preserve your sitting and standing balance through exercises designed to challenge it. I still run the risk of falling whenever my balance is challenged or when my body is extremely fatigued, otherwise I am able to slowly and methodically go about my day, including two or three fitness classes with a workout at my gym/health club in between. People will tell me they admire my fortitude and perseverance when they see me working out every day. It seems they don't understand that physical activity is a reward for me. I am happiest when I'm in motion!

As a certified senior fitness instructor, I know the importance of including exercises to improve balance in my classes. I'm rewarded whenever a senior pupil tells me they are walking or sitting/standing with more confidence. As a brain injury survivor with balance issues of my own, I cannot do many of the balance exercises that other personal trainers can demonstrate. I can however, get my classes to stand from a seated position, then sit back down and maintain a good posture throughout.

Try it yourself. See how many times you can stand up and sit back down while keeping your chest up, back straight and all of your core muscles held tight. Depending on how many times you do this, it can burn some calories while helping your balance at the same time.

Over the years, my therapists have given me many invaluable exercises to improve my balance. The trick is to actually do them. Just knowing about them will not improve your balance. How many times have I heard, "Practice, practice, practice?" Since I abhor having an imbalanced body, I should be diligent about doing my daily balance exercises, but I'm not. I always make time for strength and cardio exercises because I see the results of those. But balance? I know, I know … practice, practice, practice!

Chances are that those reading this chapter have better balance and mobility than I do. Remember that my imbalance is from an injured brain. I can sometimes trick my injured brain with my strong muscles, though. Now hear what Alison Cardoza, ACSM-certified personal trainer shares with her able-bodied clients.

Alison Cardoza, ASCM-Certfied Personal Trainer:

My goal as a certified personal trainer is to change lives for the better.

Cardiovascular exercise and strength training are incredibly important for the body; however, balance and coordination are possibly even more valuable. We often forget the importance of testing our balance and challenging ourselves with balance exercises. Many of us believe that if our body is not working up a sweat, why partake in such an activity?

I cannot reiterate enough the importance of incorporating balance exercises into your strength training and cardio routines. I work in a facility that serves people who are predominately 60 and older. As we age, our muscles can atrophy, and bone mass density can decrease. Falls occur. Bones can break.

Many of my clients suffer from osteoporosis. My goal is to increase their strength, but also to improve their coordination and balance to prevent a fall or a broken bone. Taking that initiative to challenge my clients with a balance exercise daily will improve their coordination and decrease their chances of falling and injuring a joint.

My favorite balance exercises consist of the Tight Rope Walk, the Grapevine, the Flamingo, and the balance board.

Let's start with the "Tight Rope Walk." The tight rope walk consists of walking a straight line, one foot in front of the other. Many laugh and refer to this exercise as the "sobriety test." Walking a straight line is more difficult than you may imagine. Good posture, shoulders rolled back and focusing on a spot as one walks are very important. Breathing in through the nose and out through the mouth while walking the straight line keeps the oxygen flowing and helps one relax. I start my clients off with 10 to 20 steps depending on their level. The next day we do this same exercise again, adding on more steps to complete. I like to refer to the 1 to 5 number scale when challenging my clients. 1=easy, to 5=most challenging. I encourage them to express their level of difficulty with me so we can start slowly and work each session on improving their balance. Realistic, small, reachable goals are what we aim to achieve.

The Grapevine is a great coordination and balance exercise. This exercise should be performed slowly and in a controlled manner. I will have my clients step to the side with one foot, and the other foot will follow behind and then in front, creating a weaving motion. I will encourage my clients to travel one direction for 30 seconds and then change directions. If my clients struggle with this exercise, I allow them to hold onto a ballet bar to help control their balance until practice makes perfect and they advance to just fingertips on the bar, then advance to no longer needing the ballet bar.

The Flamingo is a fun way to envision yourself as a beautiful pink bird standing on one leg! My clients use a ballet bar to hold onto if need be. If they feel this exercise is difficult, and they rank it a #5, we use the ballet bar. If it is challenging, but I feel they do not need assistance, I persuade my clients to stand on one straight leg, the other bent at the knee, with no assistance. I test them and see how long they can balance on one foot. Each session, I add on more seconds. Their balance will improve each time because their confidence, security and awareness are heightened. They focus on a particular spot and keep their abdomen engaged. Visualize a string attached to your head pulling you up to the ceiling. This visualization will help your posture and improve balance.

Balance boards are a great way to challenge the strength in the foot and ankle. My clients step on the board and try to maintain a steady balance. Again, the key is to focus on a spot and not take your eyes off. Many of my clients refer to this exercise as the surf board. The rocking back-and-forth motion resembles surfing in the ocean. Believe it or not, this exercise can prevent many falls from occurring. How many times do we say, "That curb came out of nowhere!" or "I did not see that last step?" The balance board can help us recover quickly and regain balance without falling.

Testing your balance is the first step. Practicing and actively challenging yourself daily will prevent falls and improve your overall coordination. Falls can cause injury and loss of mobility. Take care of your joints and practice balance exercises daily. Try incorporating the "Flamingo" while you prepare dinner, or while brushing your teeth. Make it a family game and see who can stand on one foot the longest! Keep it fun and save your joints by practicing these balance exercises daily!

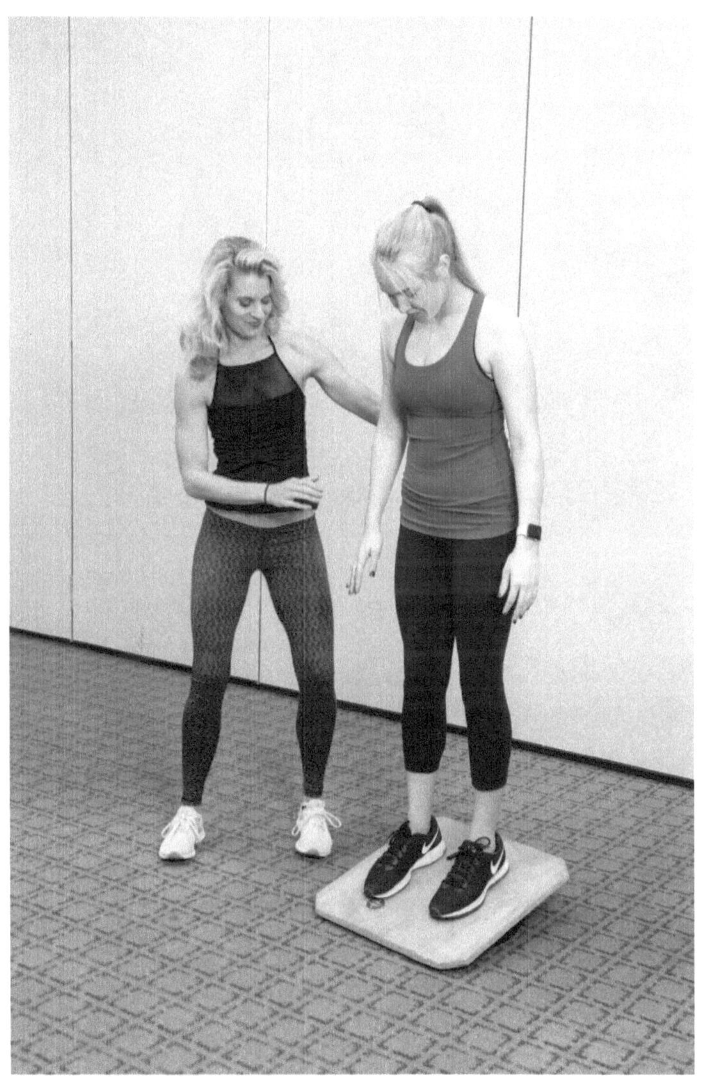

Balance board

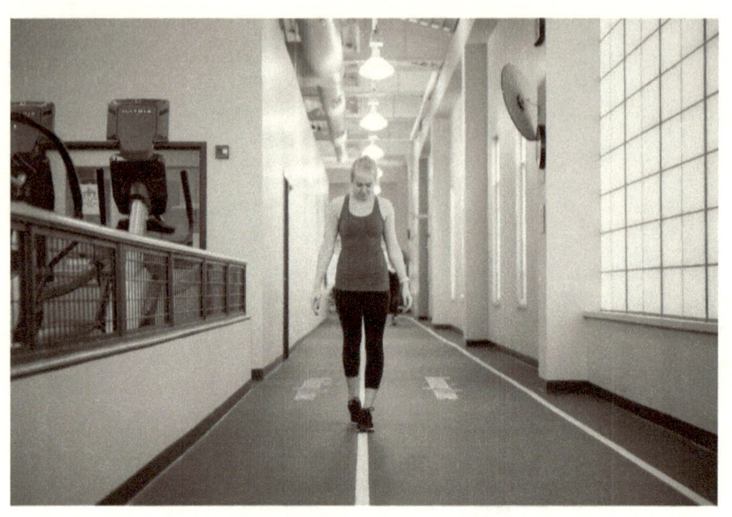

Tightrope walk

Chapter 12

Connecting Mind and Body Thru Yoga/Pilates

This will bring health to your body and nourishment to your bones.

Proverbs 3:8

At 5' 2" tall, I calculate the caloric value of everything that goes into my mouth, and estimate the number of calories I burn with every activity. I'd like to say I became a runner because I wanted to be healthier, with a better cardiovascular system. That would be a fib, though. I ran because I wanted to eat without fear of getting fat.

I remember when yoga first became popular. I tried one class, but decided I didn't have time to waste on an exercise with no aerobic potential. I wanted to burn calories! It wasn't until after my brain injury that I became a regular yoga class participant. I always stayed by the mirrored-wall with the bar so I could hang on if I needed to.

Yoga class has taught me more about how to keep my body in perfect alignment than any class I have ever taken. I still use many of the cues that my yoga instructor used in the strength and balance classes I teach at senior homes today. I get a kick out of watching the upright posture of my class change when I say the words, *'navel to spine.'*

Being flexible has, fortunately, always come naturally for me. Yoga gave me names for it! Every morning I start with, and every evening I end with *'child's pose.'* It's a wonderful way to get all the kinks out of your back.

I have to be honest and tell you that I've never taken a Pilates class. I've heard it's excellent for building a strong core. Since good core muscles are vital to maintaining good balance, you may ask why I haven't tried it. I'm embarrassed to say that I'm too much a creature of habit. Pilates has not fit into my schedule, despite its obvious benefit to me. Isn't that a little bit like all of us? Since I'm writing this book, I will make a point of taking a class now.

Now let's see what Bekki Jo, our yoga/Pilates instructor has to say about the benefits of the two and how they can fit into the fitness routine of those with chronic conditions.

I have been a fitness professional for 28 years. I began in the fitness industry as a step instructor and personal trainer. I was one of those people who would go the hardest, jump the highest and hang on for the longest. Today, my fitness world is very different. Most of my personal workouts are done in the HOT YOGA studio, BARRE studio or PILATES studio. I am currently a Pilates Reformer Trainer and BARRE/Yoga Instructor for Baptist Health Milestone Wellness Center in Louisville, Kentucky. I teach about ten BARRE or Yoga group classes per week and train approximately 35 clients per week. I offer FREE 30 minute demonstrations on the Pilates Reformers in order to introduce the discipline to new clients. In my 28-year career, Pilates and Yoga have created the most miraculous changes in clients who come to me with chronic issues; and by miraculous I mean substantial changes in overall health/wellness and quality of life.

I am a huge advocate of exercising the mind and body through the practice of Pilates and yoga. Both forms of exercise address the mind and muscular connection of the body. Both Pilates and yoga train the body to utilize CORE LOCK (mula bonda) or pelvic floor contraction to create greater strength, balance, and endurance in the muscular system. In simpler terms, I would explain this action to women as performing a "Kegel exercise," or to men as engaging the pelvic floor as if trying to stop the flow of urination. CORE LOCK is the key to CORE STRENGTH. In addition, the deep controlled breathing techniques taught in each practice are beneficial in improving lung capacity and overall respiratory health. There are many types of breathing techniques taught and they may vary from Pilates to yoga. Deep breathing and breath control are extremely important, because without oxygen we cannot live, we cannot heal and we cannot get stronger. In my group classes as well as one-on-one I concentrate on verbally cueing the deep, slow inhalations and even slower exhalations. People have a tendency to hold the breath; therefore, a constant verbal reminder is very important.

Joseph Pilates developed the Pilates Method in the 1920s and introduced his method to America in order to aid in dancer, gymnast and athlete rehabilitation. Since then, the Pilates Method has been practiced by many for several reasons: rehabilitation after various surgical procedures, chronic health issues/disease/disability, improving flexibility, and improving core strength, just to name a few.

The Pilates Method emphasizes core strength; each activity, from the warm up, to the core sequence, low back, chest/arms, and hip sequence all include intense pelvic floor contraction and core engagement. Very important for all people; but especially important for those who have chronic conditions or injuries.

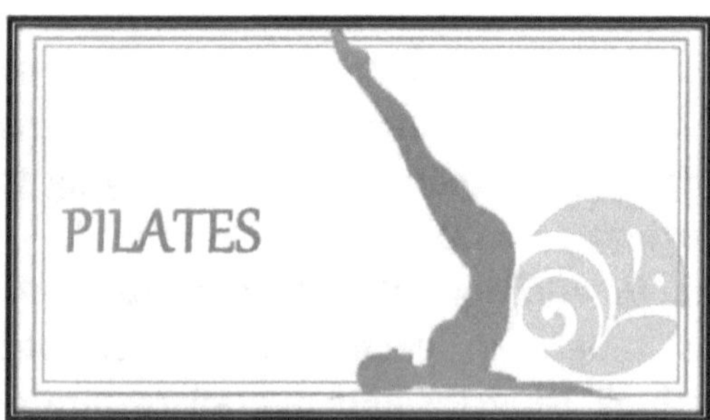

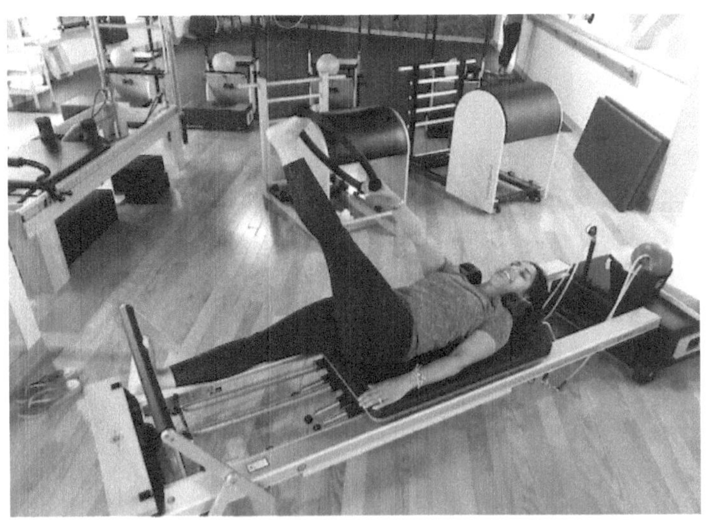

Pilates reformer

Twice a week I see Don for Pilates Reformer Training. Don has been diagnosed with chronic bulging disc in the lower lumbar spine, with three discs pushing in toward his stomach. In hopes of not having to go through surgery, Don contacted me for Pilates Reformer training. In working with Don, the first thing I noticed was that he held his breath when trying to exercise. This concept is known as the Valsalva Maneuver. This would cause him to strain, grunt, groan, sweat a lot, strain and pull muscles and fatigue quickly. For Don, I found it important to help him learn to take deep breaths. He seemed as if his lung capacity was hindered and as if he had been shallow breathing for most of his life. We spent the greater part of his first class package learning how to take deep breaths in through the nose and out through the nose. In yoga, this form of breathing is called UJJAYI (ooh-JAH-yee) breathing. This form of PRANAYAMA, or breathing exercise, is used to calm the mind and warm the body. In addition it brings presence and awareness. Through practiced deep breathing exercise, Don has been better able to oxygenate his body, warm his body and create a better mind-body connection. While learning proper breathing techniques, Don has been better able to strengthen his core muscles, allowing him to relieve much of his lower lumbar back pain. Ujjayi breathing is NOT normally a PRANAYAMA that I would teach in Pilates simply because Ujjayi is more of a meditative and warming breath and more appropriate for yoga. However, Don really needed to learn how to take DEEPER, more controlled breaths, and Ujjayi seemed to work best for him.

There are THREE breathing patterns that are taught more in Pilates training to help control the breathing pattern and to make sure that body is fully oxygenated during the exercises: LATERAL BREATHING, SET BREATH PATTERNS and ACTIVE BREATHING.

LATERAL BREATHING concentrates on the lateral expansion of the rib cage with a constant contraction of the PELVIC FLOOR and RECTUS ABDOMINIS (up and down muscles of the abdominals) during the inhalation and the exhalation of the breath. This is commonly coached in class as deep controlled breaths and zipping the abdominals up and in. This is the preferred method of breathing during Pilates.

SET BREATH PATTERNS are commonly used in Pilates as well. The inhalation happens during one movement and the exhalation happens during the second phase of the movement; commonly coached as one breath, one movement. In coaching SET BREATH PATTERNS, the client is less likely to hold the breath.

ACTIVE BREATHING is used during very specific Pilates exercises where a more forceful breath is necessary. For example, a Pilates Hundred calls for four counts breathing in and four counts breathing out, with each breath recruiting a tighter contraction of the core. The breath is usually sharper and more forceful, also recruiting the intercostal muscles which are located in the chest walls and attached to the ribs and help increase and decrease breath volume during exercise.

Some of the main benefits of PILATES and YOGA are:

It is an invigorating mind-body workout, which is extremely important for those with chronic conditions. It allows the mind to concentrate on the action at hand, allowing for mental relaxation.

It develops a strong core (strong abdominals and lower back). Core strength is the key to all activities; therefore, it is extremely important for athletic activities, but also for the daily routine (sitting, standing and mobility).

Recently, I had one of my long-time clients, Tom, write a brief testimonial for my social media campaign. This is what he said:

"I have been doing Pilates at Milestone for six years, which has strengthened my abdominal area, resulting in less pressure and pain in my lower back. Bekki Jo is a certified Pilates instructor who has worked with me to lessen my lower back pain through a variety of strengthening and stretching exercises. Pilates is not for everyone, but Pilates has decreased my lower back pain, and I will continue doing Pilates with Bekki Jo." *Tom M, Milestone Member.*

Pilates helps in gaining long, lean muscles. Pilates allows one to elongate and strengthen muscle, which in turn improves muscle elasticity and joint mobility. At a time when the body is dealing with chronic pain or injury, this practice is not only effective but more soothing to the body.

Lopa has been a great client who has challenged me to create an exercise program for a physically-fit person who has Autoimmune Hypothyroidism, which is an autoimmune disorder that causes the thyroid to underproduce certain important hormones. Over a period of time Lopa has been struggling with numerous side effects from her autoimmune disorder, such as WEIGHT GAIN, MUSCLE WEAKNESS, MUSCLE ACHES/TENDERNESS/STIFFNESS, PAIN/STIFFNESS and SWELLING OF THE JOINTS. In working with her she challenges me to create effective routines for her fitness level, yet which are soothing and healing for her muscles and joints. In our routines, Lopa practices a lot of single leg and single arm activities, forcing her pelvic floor and core muscles to work hard to keep her body stabilized while elongating, stretching and increasing the elasticity of her muscles. Pilates also allows for specific leg, hip and pelvic stretches that have helped Lopa to find that balance between strength and ease that she is looking for to help her overall health and wellness.

Pilates and yoga help teach the body efficiency. Because Pilates and Yoga train the muscles to work synergistically (more than one muscle group working at a time), recruiting your core muscles to assist the body's normal muscular function creates more balance and ease for the body.

I currently have a client that I work with named Ann. She and her husband combined have lost and kept off over 200 pounds. This alone is a great feat. Ann had a stroke several years ago and has changed the way she lives, communicates and moves. In meeting Ann, I learned that she was having a bit of trouble walking and was experiencing a bit more instability in her legs than normal. I invited Ann in for a free 30-minute demonstration on the Pilates Reformer. Ann agreed and we set the appointment.

I was excited to introduce Ann to Pilates. I was more than certain it would help her in many ways. I began the demonstration as I normally would. Ann and I did not get off on the right foot. I felt she was not following what I was asking her to do and I could not figure out what to do or say differently. I stopped our demonstration, and had Ann sit up and talk with me a little bit more in depth. In asking Ann a few questions she disclosed to me a few things that would help me better communicate with her. She told me since she had her stroke she does not respond well to multiple commands at once, nor does she respond to numbers. This changed everything. I was able to create commands that were simple and easy for her to understand, which also allowed for me to synergize movement without stressing her out with multiple commands.

Being able to communicate with Ann the way her brain allows her to communicate has not only enlightened me as a fitness professional but it has allowed me to create a Pilates-oriented fitness program that has helped Ann to get stronger in the areas that she was struggling in: her leg strength, core strength and balance, and enhance her awareness in other areas, such as deep breathing and pelvic floor connect.

Pilates and yoga help prevent injury. Because Pilates and yoga help strengthen, stretch and create flexibility and mobility in the small and large muscle groups, the tendons and ligaments are in turn strengthened to help prevent injury and improve overall health. This aspect is extremely important to the seasoned athlete, but almost more important to those dealing with chronic issues.

When I am teaching ANY type of fitness class, but most importantly Pilates and Yoga, I coach my students to listen to their bodies when exercising. Exercise in itself is self-care; however, we can still care for ourselves when we are exercising. Pilates and Yoga is a lot less intense on the body when it comes to impact and over-exertion. Pilates and Yoga can be designed for everybody, and every body can adjust and enjoy the benefits of injury prevention and self-care.

I am available at Baptist Health Milestone Wellness Center Monday thru Friday. I can be reached at bekkijo33@gmail.com or on Instagram at bekkitressler. I would be happy to help you through your fitness journey in any way possible.

<u>**Other Resources**</u>

Hypothyroidism, <u>mayoclinic.org</u>, 1999-2018

Mayo Foundation for Medical Education and Research

How to Practice Ujjayi Breath in Today, <u>YogaOutlet.com</u>

Pilates Anatomy, Rael Isacowitz and Karen Clippinger, "Learn three ways to control breathing during Pilates. <u>humankenetics.com</u>

Benefits of Pilates, <u>Pilates.com</u>

Chapter 13

Without Good Bones … You Don't Have a Leg to Stand On

The righteous person may have many troubles, but the Lord delivers him from them all; he protects all his bones, not one of them will be broken.

Psalm 34:19,20

I began having issues with my bone density even before the Baby Boomers turned 60 years old and the media overflowed with information about good bone health.

My traumatic brain injury was in 1997, when I was 37 years old. Prior to that, I had been a long-distance runner for 15 years. Poor balance was the most obvious manifestation of my brain injury, so running quickly became a thing of the past. Walking with assistance became my new normal.

I slipped one day in the bathroom and broke my ankle. My sister-in-law, Kim, who was also my gynecologist, had the good sense to order a bone scan. I was diagnosed with osteopenia, meaning I had low bone mineral density. It was a warning sign that I was on my way to osteoporosis.

I was confused. How can a distance runner and weight lifter end up with osteopenia? Kim explained that being flat on my back the 6-8 weeks I was in a coma had caused it. I was active before my accident. This new diagnosis propelled me to move even more. I teach fitness classes twice a day, five days a week. I do strength training twice or usually three times a week. I sometimes think I may exercise too much.

Daily calcium supplements plus a calcium-replacement injection every six months have kept my bone density at the same level, or slightly improved, since my osteopenia diagnosis. If I continue my strength training, surely I can avoid osteoporosis.

Now let's read what Dena Mullen, Physical Therapist, has to tell us about keeping your bones strong.

Dena Mullin, Physical Therapist

Osteoporosis is a disease that can have a significant impact on aging Baby Boomers in their later years. As we get older, there is an increased risk for fall-related fractures due to decreased bone density or thickness. There are some frightening statistics associated with osteoporosis. In the U.S. today, 54 million individuals are estimated to already have

osteoporosis or low bone mass, and approximately 50% of women and up to 25% of men will fracture a bone due to osteoporosis.

Osteoporosis is a silent disease with no symptoms, often not detected until you get a fracture. Oftentimes you could have other illnesses along with osteoporosis, which can decrease how long you live, lower your quality of life, and possibly lead to long-term nursing care in a nursing home. Osteoporosis is more often seen in women of European origin (Caucasian) and in women with low body weight and height; however, osteoporosis is affecting men and people of other ethnicities as well.

Osteoporosis is a disease that affects our bones. Bone is a living, growing tissue that is constantly changing. Osteoporosis can cause your bone to become porous and honeycomb-like—less dense. Your bone is made mostly of collagen—a protein that provides the soft framework, and calcium phosphate—a mineral that adds strength to the framework. Our bone is formed from the time we are born and continues to build until we reach peak bone mass at the age of 30-35. We acquire 85-90% of our adult bone mass by the time we reach age 18 in girls and 20 in boys.

Osteoporosis is caused by loss of our bone, a change in our bone structure, and is characterized by low bone mass and structural deterioration of bone tissue. Our adult skeletal system is maintained through the process of bone remodeling and resorption. The process of bone remodeling—bone formation or bone building, and bone resorption, or bone breakdown and loss, occurs throughout life. Bone remodeling is a delicate balance between **resorption** and redeposition of bone mineral, which can eventually lead to osteoporosis. As we age, this balance changes and our bones can become porous, brittle, and fragile, causing fractures to occur without trauma or minimal injury. Osteoporosis leads to bone fragility and increases your risk of fractures of the hip, spine and wrist. Fall-related fractures and those due to weak, brittle bones could increase morbidity (your quality of health and well being) and mortality (your risk for death) as well as the psychosocial impact of fear of repeated falls and loss of independence.

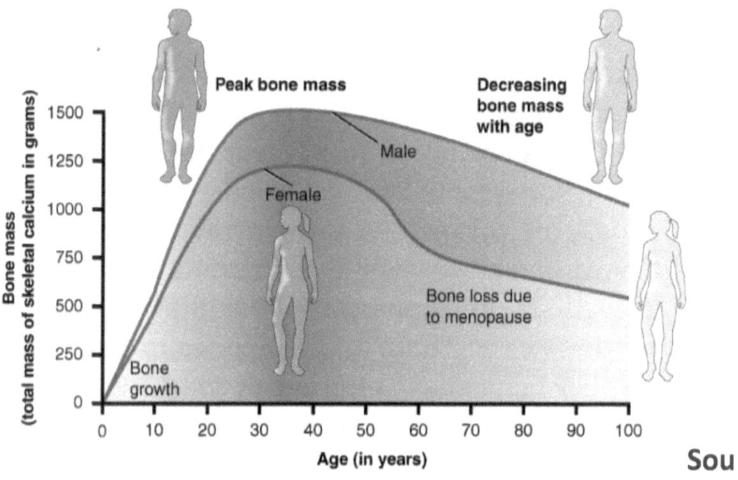

Source: http://www.primarycareutah.com/bone-density-testing

Osteoporosis Risk Factors

You have some risk factors that are not controllable. You cannot control your gender or age. Being female and more than 50 years old increases your risk of acquiring osteoporosis. For most women, bone loss increases after menopause by as much as 20% or more of their bone density. Other uncontrollable risk factors include low body mass index or weight, stature or posture, being post-menopausal, and if you have a family history of osteoporosis. Being female and over 50 years old is considered the greatest uncontrollable risk factor. There are other medical conditions that you need to consider that can increase your risk of osteoporosis. These medical conditions include diabetes, menopause, rheumatoid arthritis, chronic gastrointestinal diseases, chronic obstructive pulmonary disease, thyroid disease and the use of medications such as corticosteroids, thyroid medication, anticonvulsants, anticoagulants, antacids with aluminum, and diuretics.

Fortunately there are risk factors that you can control. These controllable risk factors include diet, lifestyle, use of tobacco, alcohol, and caffeine, and weight control. You need to have an active lifestyle that includes exercise, at least three times a week. Exercise can decrease the amount of bone loss and actually stimulates the formation of new bone! Smoking decreases estrogen production and smoking, alcohol, and caffeine interfere with calcium absorption. As you age you should be taking calcium and vitamin D supplements to help with bone loss, and the Vitamin D can also help with balance. Another controllable risk is eating disorders. Make sure to eat a healthy diet rich in calcium-enriched foods. Also be aware of any fall risks in your home as well as outside your home.

Most osteoporosis education is directed at the 65-year old female of European descent. There is limited awareness of the impact of osteoporosis on women of color and men. Women of color, including African-Americans and Hispanics, and men, often believe they are free from osteoporosis risk. If you are a woman or man of color you need to be aware that up to 75% of African-American women and men are lactose intolerant and should avoid consuming dairy products in their bone-building years from childhood to young adulthood. The National Institutes of Health report the risk of death following a hip fracture for African-American women is more likely than for Caucasian women. Diseases such as sickle-cell anemia and lupus can further increase the risk of developing osteoporosis in the African-American population. In all age groups, Hispanic women typically consume less than the recommended dietary allowance of calcium, with 10% of Hispanics over the age of 50 being osteoporotic, and 49% of that age group is diagnosed with osteopenia.

If you are a man, you are not safe from osteoporosis. The statistics for men acquiring osteoporosis are also significant. In men over the age of 50, 1 in 4 will fracture a bone due to osteoporosis. Did you know that older men have a greater chance of getting an osteoporotic fracture than developing prostate cancer? Also, older men are more likely to die within the 1st year following a hip fracture compared to women; and, by the age of 65-70, men have an equal risk of osteoporosis to that of women. These are frightening statistics!

People of color and men are underserved and undereducated in osteoporosis awareness, education and prevention. Women of color believe they are protected by their ethnicity, and men believe they are protected by their gender. If you are in one of these groups, being identified as to your susceptibility to high risk of fracture is crucial to high quality of life in your later years. Both of these groups need advocacy for improved evaluation and assessment for the development of osteoporosis.

How do I know if I have osteoporosis?

The best way to identify if you have osteoporosis or are at risk is via a DXA scan. The World Health Organization (WHO) categorizes osteoporosis based on the measurement of bone mineral density (BMD) via central dual-energy X-ray absorptiometry (DXA) to establish or confirm a diagnosis of osteoporosis and to predict your future risk of a fracture. DXA is the gold standard diagnostic test in the diagnosis of osteoporosis prior to the occurrence of a fracture. In postmenopausal women and in men aged 50 and older, WHO diagnostic T-score criteria are applied to BMD at the lumbar spine and femoral neck as follows: a T-score of -2.5 or below standard deviation of the reference BMD for young adults is a diagnosis of osteoporosis and a T-score between 1 to 2.5 standard deviation below the reference is osteopenia.

http://www.naturalhealthadvisory.com/daily/osteoporosis-prevention-and-treatment/bone-density-chart-understand-your-bone-density-scores//SourSour

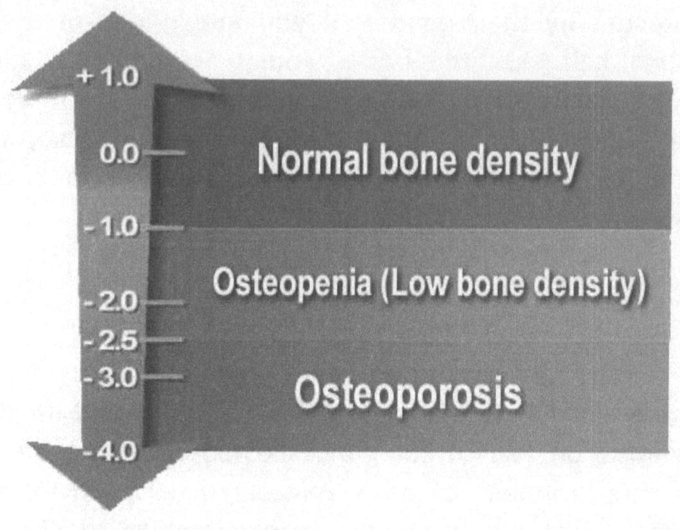

Source:
http://www.naturalhealthadvisory.com/daily/osteoporo
sis-prevention-and-treatment/bone-density-chart-
understand-your-bone-density-scores/

How do I keep my risk as low as possible?

The steps for keeping healthy bones and slowing the progression of osteoporosis include: eating a healthy diet rich in calcium and vitamin D; exercising at least three times a week with emphasis on weight bearing and strengthening exercises; maintaining a healthy lifestyle which excludes smoking and excessive alcohol consumption; and having bone density testing and medications when appropriate to increase the rate of bone tissue formation.

When looking for osteoporosis exercise programs there are important components that should be included in the exercise program. These components are: adherence to an exercise program; weight bearing exercises for maintaining or improving BMD; spinal stabilization and strengthening exercises; postural and body mechanics exercises; and balance exercises for fall prevention.

The great news is that osteoporosis can be prevented in most people. The best defense is to build strong bones before age 30 and maintain a healthy lifestyle. There is only treatment to prevent further demineralization of bones. Prevention is the key because currently there is no cure for osteoporosis.

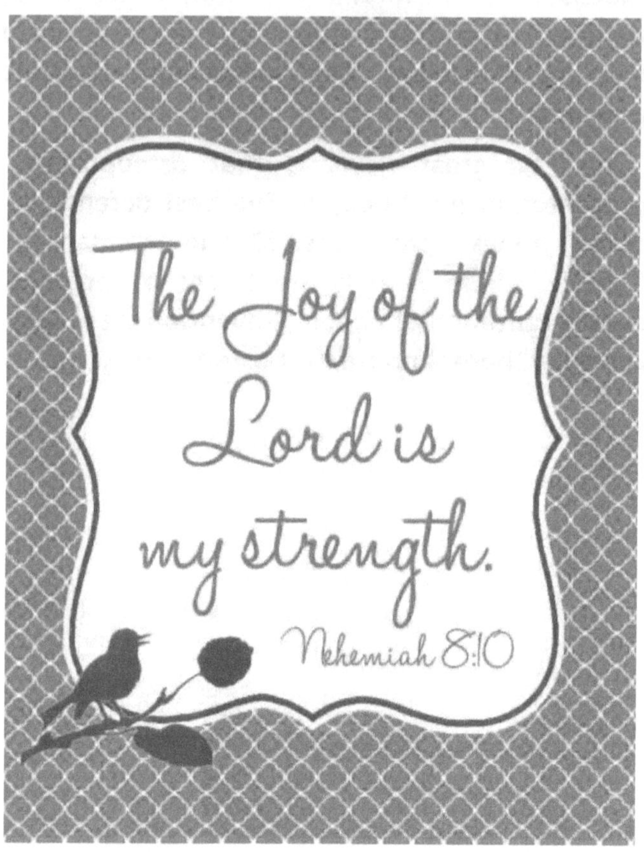

The Joy of the Lord is my strength.
Nehemiah 8:10

Chapter 14

Healing Waters

Now the earth was formless and empty, darkness was over the surface of the deep, and the Spirit of God was hovering over the waters.

Genesis 1:2

A few months after my brain injury, I went to visit my cousins in Naples, Florida. The vacation home we rented had an indoor pool. It was then I realized I could walk very carefully with no support. Chest-level water made me very buoyant. I would walk and walk and walk, only to be frustrated when I crumbled again on dry ground.

I didn't get back in a pool for a few years after that. Then my physical therapist, Dena, got me in the therapy pool (It's warm!) at my health club, Baptist Milestone. Dena put a flotation device around my waist and attached it to the side of the pool with a long tube. Then she told me to start running. I was scared at first, but soon I was lifting my knees and pumping my arms like I was in a 10K race! I loved it, but never did it again. I was, and still am, kind of paranoid about putting people out to make me mobile.

The real truth is that I like my workouts to be quick, without a lot of preparation time. Pool time requires extra clothes, towels and being extra cautious not to slip. I really do feel like I'm working my muscles better in water, but there are only so many hours in a day. Every time I'm in the pool, I tell myself I'm going to start coming regularly.

Maybe Zorré Kimura can sell me on the concept. Z is a physical therapist who spends a lot of time in the water with his patients.

By Zorré Z. Kimura, PT, DPT

In the beginning and until our last days, water makes up a significant part of our bodies. Our life is dependent on the water we drink, and without hydration our cells and organs cease to function. For many people with painful joints or painful muscle tissue, the thought of living without water in the form of aquatic exercise would seem like a sentence to the pain prison!

For those of you who have found bliss in the spirit of the water, this chapter is truly preaching to the choir. But this chapter is really for those who are searching for a better way to move. For some reason, many of you reading this book find water intimidating, or not worth the time it takes to change, shower, etc. So you keep on

wondering about exercising in water, wondering if you should give it a try. For others, you've tried exercising in the pool but found it ineffective, or even to have increased your pain.

I'm a physical therapist and some people call me Dr. Z. At least the students do where I'm on faculty in the Doctorate PT program here in Louisville. Most of my patients over the past 36 years have just called me Z.

Growing up in Hawaii from the age of 3 established my love for water from the beginning. But my love for the water also comes with quite a bit of respect, due to a near drowning while surfing at the age of 16, and then at 19 a surfing injury that tore cartilage in my knee. That surgery had a major impact on my life and recently led to a total knee replacement at the age of 57.

Water helped me get better at 19. First the pool, then back to the beach where I walked in the sand, swam, and then buried my knee in the sand to reduce swelling (an ancient Hawaiian trick that really works). Eventually I returned to running, tennis, teaching aerobics, and other impact sports that in retrospect I should not have pursued so intensely. As a physical therapist one of my first education courses was to get certified to be an aquatic exercise instructor. In my 30s I helped athletes in deep-water pools get back to sports. In my 50s here at our Wellness Center, I've helped a variety of patients understand how to get the most out of using the healing properties of water.

So what is so special about water and why is it worth the time and energy and possible bad hair for the rest of the day? I think the answers lie in two opposing forces: 1) The properties of lift or buoyancy; and 2) The properties of matter or resistance.

When I nearly drowned on that big surf day on the North Shore, I experienced one force that almost killed me, then another that saved me (plus some divine intervention). The power of matter and resistance pulled me down under the water when wave came after wave and then with my board attached to my ankle, I was like a rag doll pulled to the bottom. After what seemed like minutes in the dark abyss, I was lifted to the top, to the light, where my buoyancy and the salt-water buoyancy helped me find air again.

Just to be clear, this is not the story I typically tell to my patients, especially ones that have a significant fear of water. But many patients who struggle with getting into water to a depth of at least chest high, have a story to tell about why they've shied away from aquatic exercise or therapy. Many just grew up where learning to swim was limited due to a lack of available or affordable pools. Some of my patients, however, tell stories of being introduced to swimming by being thrown into the deep end. Well-meaning, or maybe just mean, friends and relatives tossed these patients into pools or ponds thinking that the freestyle or breaststroke would just come "naturally" to these folks. After coughing and crying and years of anxiety, many patients come to our aquatic PT program terrified, and understandably so.

So back to the principles and how we apply them to each of our patients.

Buoyancy

In physics, buoyancy, or upthrust, is an upward force exerted by a fluid that opposes the weight of an immersed object.[1] More simply, one's ability to float depends on factors like depth of water and the density of the patient/swimmer.

Our focus when it comes to "unloading" the spine or joints at the hip or knee is based on finding the right water depth, and sometimes we have to add additional floating devices to increase buoyancy. These extra devices are usually foam-based and can be in the water shoes that people wear, foam noodles of various sizes, jogging-type belts fastened at the waist, or different sizes of foam dumbbells.

The first goal with this principle in mind is to find your depth plus float device (if necessary) to allow you to move with the safest amount of impact on your joints. This may range anywhere from no impact in the deepest end of the pool plus floats, belts, and shoes to standing in water from stomach height to the level of the collar bone. Deeper water is often better for patients with severe osteoarthritis of the hip and knee, back pain due to spinal stenosis, or post-operative weight-bearing restrictions. Or, one can exercise with no added flotation in shallower water depths. In general, a good reference point for depth is water right at the mid-chest or sternum. (see picture)

It doesn't take much to flare a painful joint or lower back when the effects of gravity and body weight are not properly reduced via the physics of unloading. It's exciting to be able to move with less pain in the water. I often will spend hours in the pool in a day exercising along with patients; walking, jogging, and doing moderate to light impact work on my joints. Most days I feel pretty good at the end of the day, but sometimes I get a little carried away, forgetting that at times the water seems to "mask" or cover the pains I feel on land.

Resistance

In fluid dynamics, drag, or fluid resistance, is a force acting opposite to the relative motion of any object moving with respect to a surrounding fluid.[2]

To me, this is where the beauty of water and science merge together and become art. It's the wonder of the school of dolphins dancing in front of your boat off the coast of Kauai. It's the power of Michael Phelps winning another gold medal.

To maintain health, we must do our best to maintain muscle mass. To challenge our muscular system, we must find optimal levels of resistance. How does this look in the pool or ocean? Once again, depth plays a role in modifying resistance to the level of pain-free exercise. Movement near the surface of the water provides less drag vs. action at lower depths. Just think of water as being more like air, the closer it is to air.

The next principle for resistance is the matter of speed. While exercising quickly out of water seems to lessen resistance via momentum, speed in the water creates more opposing forces. The powerful kicks and strokes of a swimmer create speed via force, but it also depends on another principle of resistance, which takes us back to drag.

Varying levels of drag are created by the position of your hand/foot, or the type of exercise device you add to your hand, wrist, ankle, or foot. Many of the tools for drag (like foam dumbbells), are still around from the 1980s, but in the past few years, companies have created ankle straps and hand-held plastic dumbbells with high tech "blades" and "baffles." [3]

When it comes to challenging or treating a patient with a pain syndrome like fibromyalgia, choosing the right piece of equipment can mean the difference between feeling a lot better, or spending 3 days in bed with a major setback. For someone just trying to get stronger or burn calories to lose weight, not having enough resistance can lead to nothing to show but fingers wrinkled like prunes.

In summary, depth, speed and drag are keys to optimal aquatic rehab and resistive exercises. Combine that with setting yourself up in the right part of the pool based on your height, weight, and need for joint unloading, and you will optimize the principles of buoyancy. If you've got this figured out, you're on your way to a lifetime of fun and fitness. Not sure how to implement these concepts? Give your local PT or personal trainer a call. [4]

I hope I've given you some guidance for those wanting to get started. For those in the "aquatic choir," keep singing the praises of water but remember to listen to your body outside the water. If pain is talking to you, spend some time unloading. If it's getting harder to lift and push and play like you used to, consider adding more resistance to your routine. Either way, learn how to move at the speed of water, which is uniquely different for each one of us.

1, 2. Wikipedia

3. Check out equipment options at aqualogixfitness.com, San Diego, California.

4. Frequency, duration, intensity, and the type of aquatic exercise program you start with is dependent on many variables. Even the most detailed chapter dedicated to this subject would still require a disclaimer due to so many individual variables. Our patients require evaluations before we even start, and our personal trainers spend a good deal of time getting to know their clients. Even our group class instructors try to get to know the physical "issues" of the members in their class whenever possible. Large facilities like ours have classes dedicated to groups with similar characteristics like fibromyalgia, arthritis, post joint replacement, and multiple sclerosis.

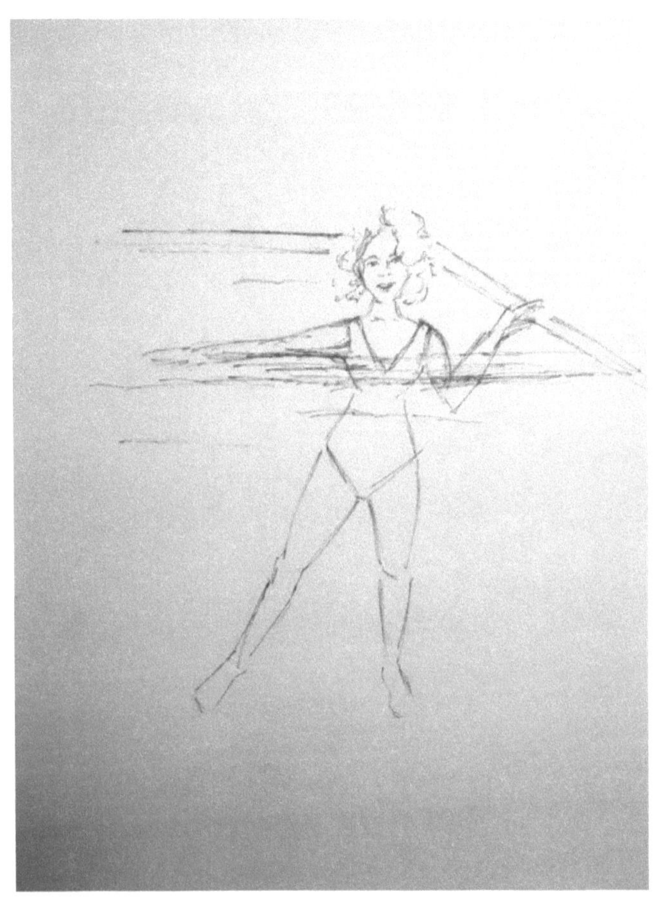

Drawing by **_Sammykimuraart.com_**

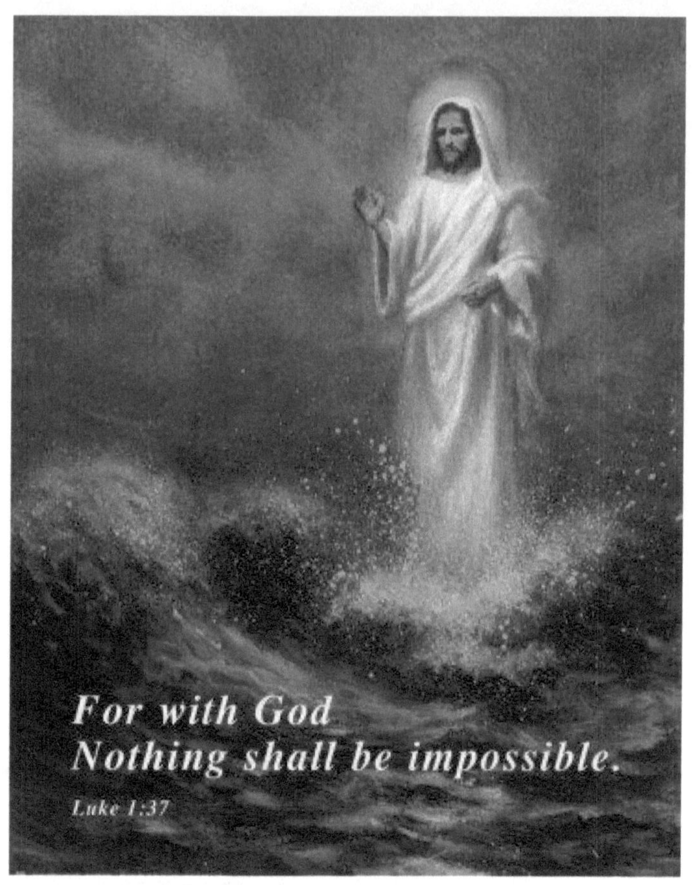
For with God
Nothing shall be impossible.
Luke 1:37

Chapter 15

Suspended Motion

I can do all this through him who gives me strength.

Philippians 4:13

TRX Suspension Training is a newer mode of exercising that I had seen at my health club and figured it was just a new craze for younger gym-goers. Remember, I'm almost an old fogey now! One day while I was doing the weight machines that I've been doing for years, I asked Jennifer, one of the personal trainers, how she managed to get her shoulders and arms so cut. You could take a pencil and trace the lines of each muscle.

I thought she was going to show me a magic weight machine. Instead, Jennifer took me into a room with numerous ropes hanging from the ceiling. She showed me how to lean back while hanging onto the ropes and do various shoulder exercises using my own body weight as resistance. I'm not buying that's the reason for her cut shoulders, but Jennifer showed me another way to keep my posture in proper alignment.

Since my balance is so poor, I innately lean slightly forward to protect it. It always feels like I'm walking with my bottom out as I lean forward. By leaning back when I grabbed the TRX ropes, my body was learning how to move using the muscles I was intending to work.

After several months of using TRX, I feel like I can walk a little more naturally. It causes me to push my hips forward, instead of sticking my bottom out. That's what the TRX Suspension Training has done for my imbalanced body. Now let's see the TRX instructor's tips for using the system with other types of chronic health conditions.

Meet Jennifer Degrella!

TRX IS SCIENTIFICALLY PROVEN TO IMPROVE TOTAL-BODY STRENGTH, STABILITY, AND EVEN CARDIOVASCULAR HEALTH. TRX HAS EMPOWERED PEOPLE OF ALL KINDS TO BE THEIR BEST VERSON OF THEMSELVES, NEVER LIMITED BY CONSTRAINTS OF TIME, PLACE, OR PHYSICAL ABILITY.

TRX is a form of suspension training that uses body-weight exercises to develop strength, balance, flexibility and core stability simultaneously. It requires the use of the TRX

Suspension Trainer, a performance training tool that leverages gravity and the user's body weight to complete the exercises.

Navy SEAL Randy Hetrick created the first version of TRX in 1997. He used a jiu-jitsu belt and parachute webbing. After Randy earned his MBA from Stanford University, he focused on developing the first version of the TRX Suspension Trainer. It was an instant hit with athletes, coaches and trainers. By 2005, TRX had more than one million users in over 60 countries.

TRX appeals to all different groups of people. It isn't limited just to young athletes. Many older adults fear falls. Those with balance and functional stability deficits may resist trying one-legged balance activities or stepping onto an unstable surface even when offered spotting help by a trainer. To lessen this fear, trainers may allow a client to grip a fixed object such as a bar or wall, which will prevent him or her from learning to use muscles to stabilize in unstable circumstances. Fortunately, when using TRX, older adults and people recovering from injuries or disabilities can try new exercises with less fear of toppling over. The device provides a dynamic point of stability, and because you're not hanging on to a fixed object you are involving core muscles and working on the large and small stability muscles. TRX is one of the most versatile pieces of equipment for the physical therapist, chiropractor, or other rehab professionals to use in the treatment of injuries as well. The exercise variety and the ease and rapidity of changing the load of the exercise makes it great for individuals of all fitness levels and ages. Introducing instability helps us engage core musculature that our beginner and/or adaptive athletes don't see on a day-to-day basis and really redefines what posture is for them.

There are seven basic movements: push, pull, plank, rotate, hinge, lunge, and squat.

PUSH (chest press)

Facing away from the anchor point, Hold the TRX handles in front of you. Brace your core and lean your weight into the handles, making sure your hips, shoulders, knees and ankles are aligned. Lower the body as your elbows bend, toward the handles. Push back to start. If this is too challenging, then offset your footing into a lunge position.

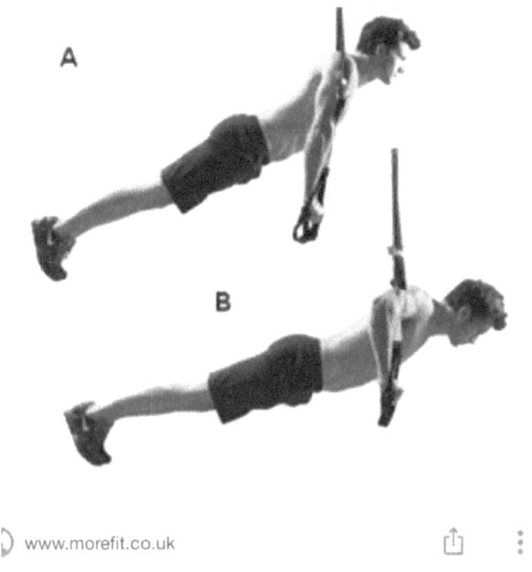

PULL (low row)

Facing the anchor, Lean back holding TRX handles. Tighten your core, with your shoulders pulled down and back. Pull your chest up to your hands, with your palms facing in. Lower yourself down in one slow, controlled movement.

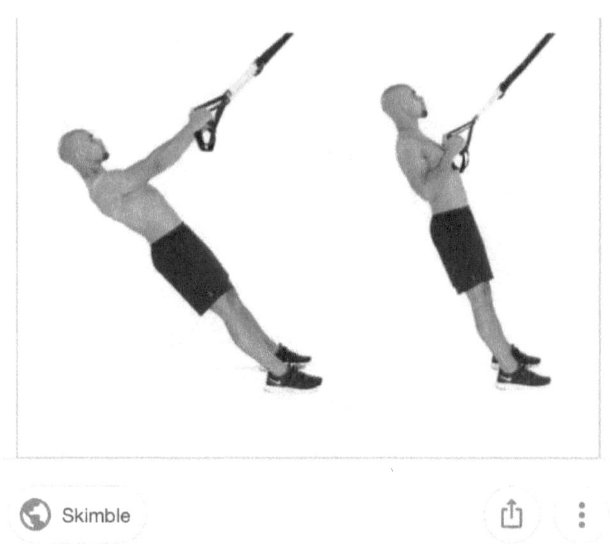

PLANK

Plank up into a pushup position, keeping your hands directly under your shoulders. Brace your core and make sure your head, shoulders, hips, knees and ankles are aligned. Lower your knees to the ground.

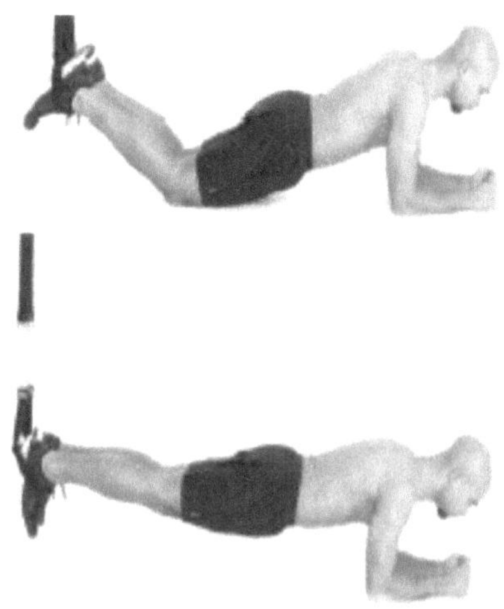

ROTATE

Place arms in a "T," body in half-kneeling position, facing away from the anchor. Maintain lengthened spine, shift hips forward, rotate torso away from rear leg, side bend away. Shift hips back to return hip to neutral, arms down.

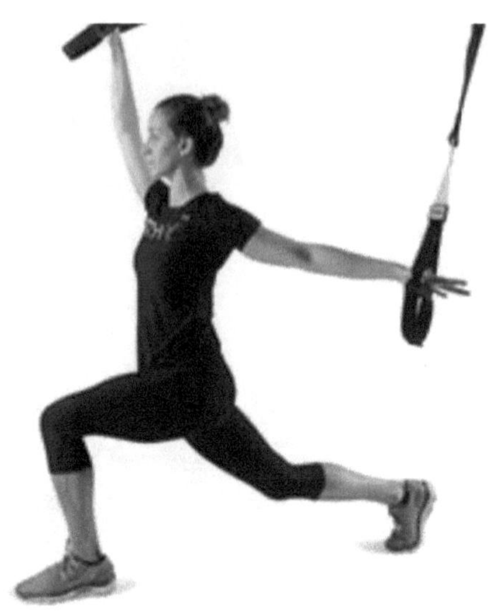

HINGE

Facing the anchor, extend arms, pressing down on handles, knees bent. Bend forward from the hips, maintain a lengthened spine, extend the knees. Press on handles, extend at hips to upright position.

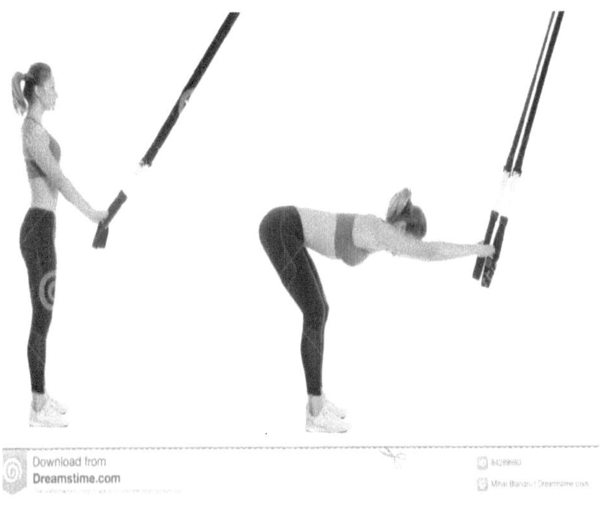

LUNGE

With one leg through both foot cradles on the TRX, ground yourself through your working leg. Push your hips down and back, and lunge down until your front knee is bent to 90 degrees. Keep your core braced and your chest up the entire time. Drive through your front foot using glute and hamstring to bring you back up.

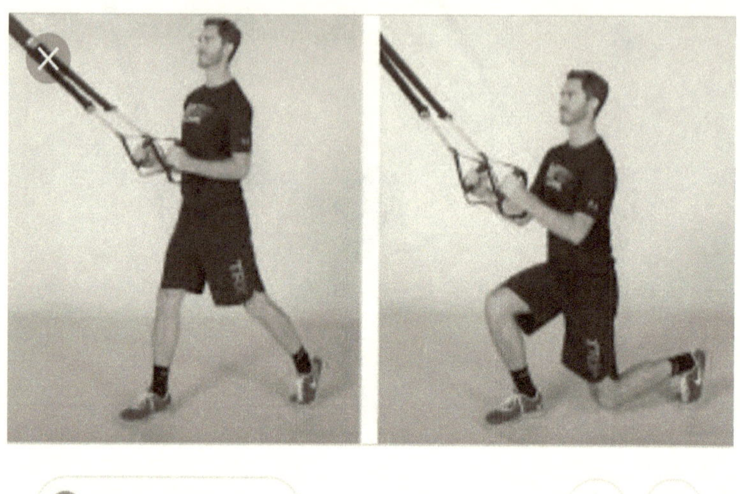

SQUAT

Stack your elbows under shoulders, with feet hip-width apart. Lower hips down and back, weight in heels. Drive through heels, squeeze glutes and lift chest.

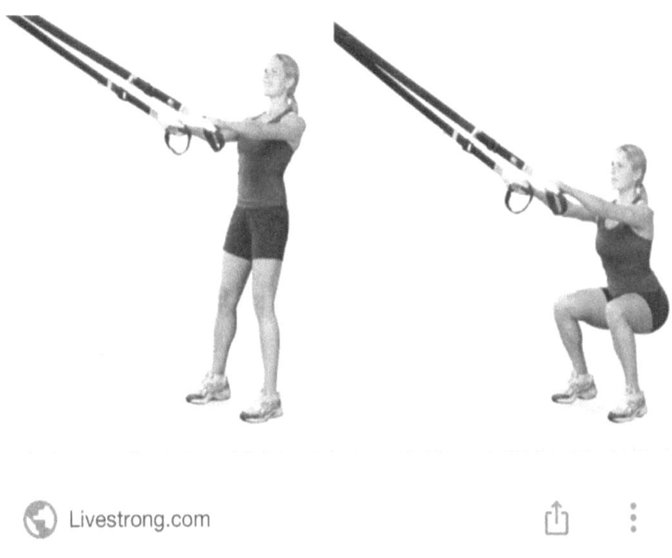

TRX training has grown in popularity over the past few years for good reason. Initially developed by the military, it has benefited athletes of all varieties from MMA and NFL to track and field. It has made its way into most gyms across the nation. While it may be intimidating at first for beginners and adaptive athletes, it is a modality that can catapult your fitness by leaps and bounds with a bit of practice and patience.

•Based on latest research and cutting-edge science: TRX training incorporates the latest fitness approaches from a variety of specialties to give you a tool that covers a multitude of training methodologies. By gathering research from the military, elite athlete training protocols, coaches and first responders, TRX allows the average gym-goer to train in a manner that exceeds what conventional gym equipment provides. It's adaptive and progressive to keep your body challenged and moving better.

•Scalable: I love a training tool that can be used by almost anyone. If you're just starting out, there are a variety of exercises you can modify to fit your fitness level. And with most of these exercises, there are small adjustments you can make to safely advance the difficulty and make progress.

•Functional: TRX training utilizes functional movement, allowing you to improve the way you move, react and perform in all areas of your life. This will translate into impressive gains in flexibility, balance, speed and strength as well.

•Core-focused: When you increase the overall strength, flexibility and endurance of your core muscles, you'll be better able to ward off injuries, perform better and achieve greater fitness results. TRX training engages your core muscles in most of the exercises due to the suspension aspect and angle of your body. You'll get a core workout without even realizing it and work muscles you never knew you had.

Static and dynamic balance play a critical role in keeping us active and injury-free. Static balance is the ability to stand in place on one leg without creating undue biomechanical stress on the body. Dynamic balance, on the other hand, is the ability of the body to maintain control over a specific base of support while in motion. Regular exercise, including balance training, ensures both static and dynamic balance get a regular workout.

The TRX Suspension Trainer is one of the most versatile and functional pieces of fitness equipment available today, requiring exercisers to leverage their own body weight against the force of gravity.

Four TRX exercises to help improve balance are:

TRX Single-Leg Hip Hinge

• Stand with the feet together, the arms reaching forward and the palms facing down.

• Hinge at the hips and load the right leg, allowing the left leg to float directly behind you until the body creates a "T" shape.

• Focus on keeping the hips square and the core strong. Try pressing down on the handles for better balance control.

Squats With Heel Raise

This classic TRX squat variation strengthens the quads and glutes and adds a balance challenge by reducing the client's base of support during the heel-raise phase.

• Stand facing the TRX anchor with the feet about hip-distance apart.

• Keeping the shoulders relaxed and chest lifted, bend at the hips and knees to lower the tailbone toward the floor.

• To stand, drive up through the heels, and then lift to balance on the balls of the feet.

• Stand tall with the arms reaching forward and the palms facing each other.

• Center the right leg to align with the TRX anchor.

• Extend the left leg behind you, and then externally rotate the leg so that the left leg crosses behind the right.

• Focus on pressing down through the right foot to maintain balance.

• Drive up through the right heel to return to the starting position.

TRX Crossing Balance Lunge

Tree Pose With Chest Stretch

This static balance exercise can be performed barefoot to improve strength in the stabilizing muscles of the foot and ankle.

• Stand holding both TRX straps while facing away from the anchor.

• Take a few steps forward to create tension on the TRX straps.

• Root the right foot into the floor while rotating the left hip open.

• The left foot may rest on the floor, inner calf or inner thigh.

• Stretch the arms out wide to a "T" or "W" position.

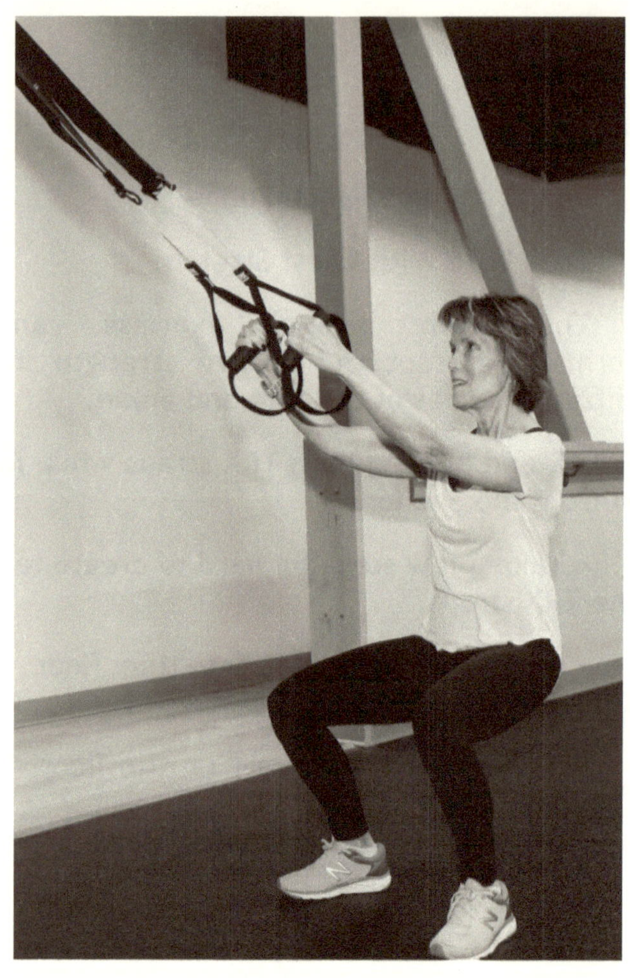

TRX squat

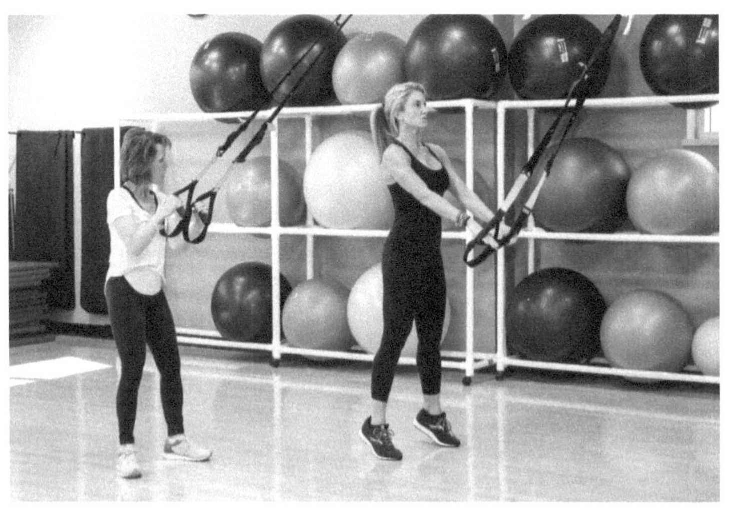

TRX Heel lifts for balance training

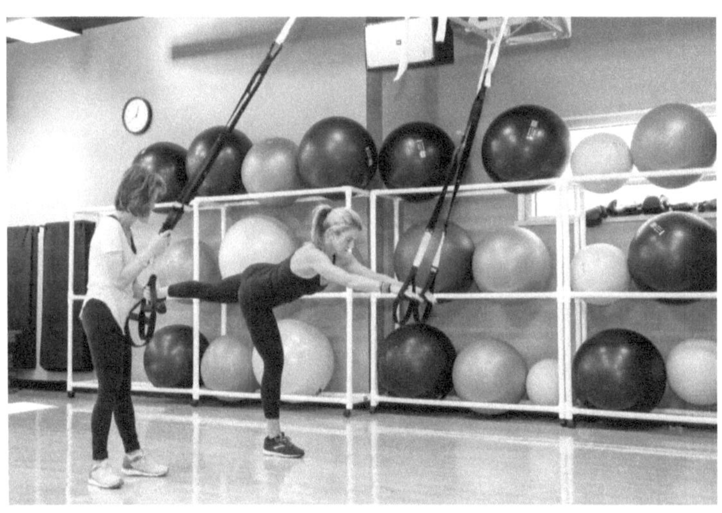

TRX Hip hinge

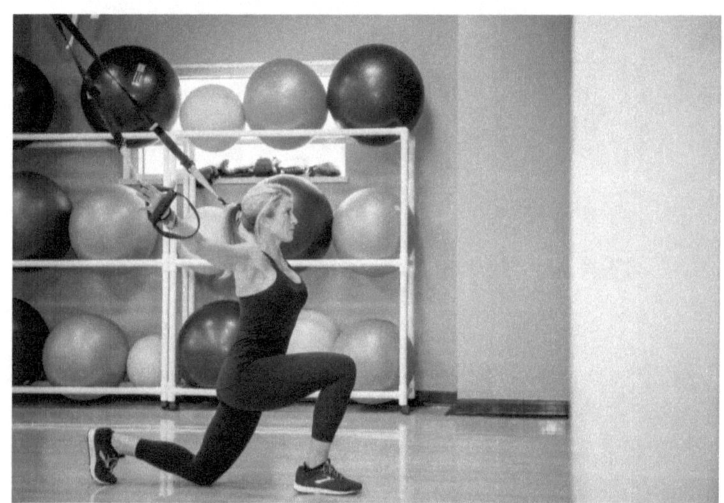

TRX lunge with fly

Chapter 16

Making the Day-to-Day Better (with Functional Training)

Whoever gives heed to instruction prospers, and blessed is the one who trusts in the Lord.

Proverbs 16:20

Because of my imbalanced body, functional training has been vital to my exercise program. I don't always do my balance exercises, but rarely does a day go by without some form of functional exercise. That's because they allow me to trick my body into feeling balanced because I engage my hip and core muscles. I can sometimes keep myself from falling by consciously tightening my core and bottom.

I will show you my three daily favorites after we hear from Mary Hayes, ACSM-Certified Personal Trainer.

Mary Hayes, ACSM-Certified Personal Trainer

What is Functional Training?

Life/Activities of Daily Living, Work, Sports

Functional training attempts to adapt or develop exercises which allow you to perform the activities of daily living, work, and/or sports more easily and without injury. Functional training aims to make your body stronger and more stable, but also more agile and flexible.

Functional training is also used in rehabilitation by physical therapists and other health experts. It is never too late to start! All adults could really benefit from starting/doing a functional training program.

Functional training is for EVERYBODY: the young, the middle-aged, or the elderly. Our muscle mass and strength will decrease 30-50% between the ages of 30-80 years old. The average person, male or female, starts losing the ability to perform everyday functions/activities of daily living as soon as they hit middle age.

In the *American Journal of Health Promotion*, a study of 87 adults aged 65-93 years old showed that functionality, or ability to move, improved for functionally-limited seniors who participated in a 16-week structured exercise program, consisting of 13 different strength-training exercises using a Thera-band resistance band.

Why functional training?

It helps our muscles to work together and prepare them for daily tasks, work, and/or sports, by simulating common movements you might use at home, work or playing a sport. Just think of all the different muscles you use and movements you make putting your groceries away. Wouldn't you like that to be easier?

Examples of functional training

Squat – It trains the muscles used when you rise up and down from a chair or pick up objects from the floor or low places.

Multi-directional lunges - help your body with balance in common activities such as vacuuming and yard work.

Push-ups - from either the floor on hands and toes OR hands and knees - strengthen the chest and shoulders for actions such as putting away items on a high shelf to pushing a grocery cart to pushing a lawn mower.

Single-leg dumbbell rows - improve hip stability, large muscles in the back, AND balance.

Toe touches - stretch out the lower back, glutes , and hamstrings.

Dumbbell shoulder press - strengthens the shoulder girdle and triceps to pick up heavy objects and to push you up out of a chair.

Using the muscles in the upper and lower body simultaneously will ignite your core strength and stability. Examples of this would be: squats with dumbbells, lunging with dumbbells.

Exercises performed sitting on a stability ball improve core and hip stability. They challenge the muscles in the lower back, hips, and quadriceps.

Planks help with all-over body strength, targeting the core.

Most fitness and training facilities now have stability balls, foam rollers, balance boards, and other tools as a part of their conditioning/functional training equipment. These are the tools of the trade!

<u>Client testimony</u>

Anne, 72, is a client I have been working with since 2013. Anne at the time had been working out and was moderately fit, but her current trainer was preparing to move out of town and asked me if I could work with her. Doing an assessment on her, we talked about goals and her physical concerns. She was having pain in her right knee and was told by her doctor that a knee replacement was in her future. I started her with functional training, strengthening, mobility, and flexibility exercises. Staying virtually pain-free, it was 3 years later that she went in for her knee replacement. Six months post-surgery, she was pain-free, going up and down the stairs, taking her dog for long walks, and back to her 4-days-a-week workout regimen, and traveling. In her words, the knee replacement AND the functional training are "the best decisions she ever made."

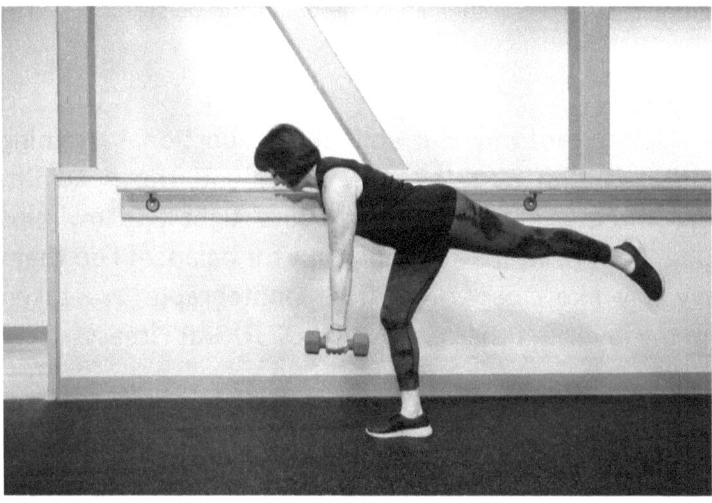

Single leg exercise with weight

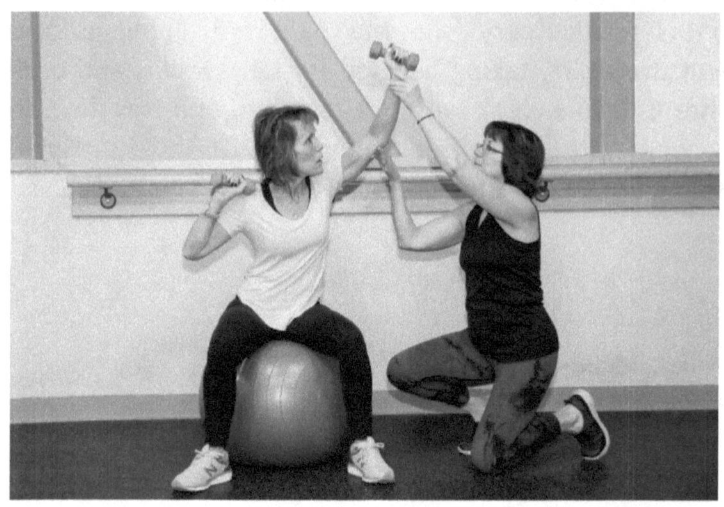

Multi-tasking? Dumbbell lift while balancing on stability ball.

Here are my current three Functional Training favorites … the bird-dog, the plank, and the dead lift. These three exercises keep my core tight and my hips strong, both of which are important for balance! I do them every day like clockwork! These photographs are taken from my favorite fitness website, POPSUGAR Fitness.

The bird-dog

This challenges my balance. I do 8-10 repetitions every morning after dressing. Then I feel like I've awakened my core and hip muscles for the day.

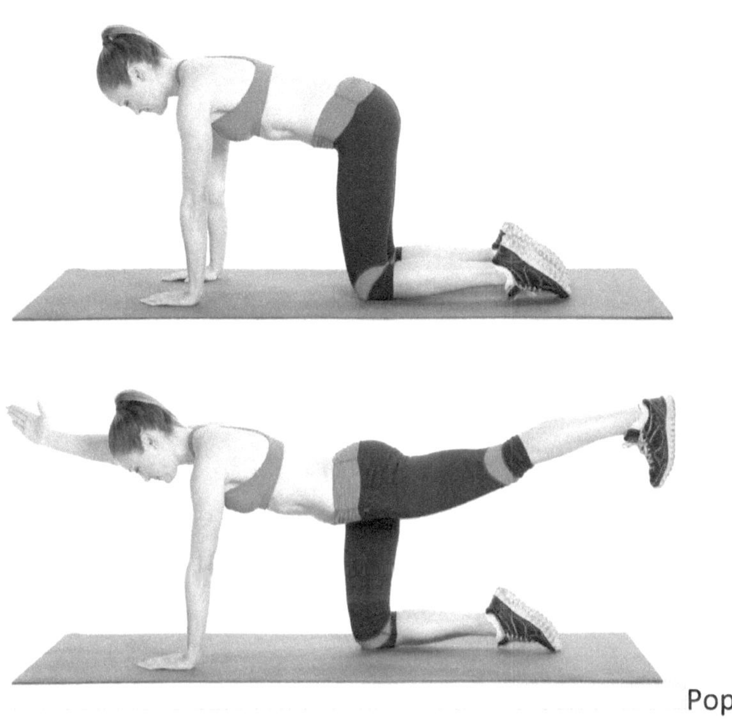

Sugar Fitness.com

Start by kneeling on all fours. Then extend opposite arm/leg straight in front and behind you. To maintain my balance I concentrate on pushing my hip bone forward and up. Keep your core muscles tight and your chest elevated. Then count, "One-one thousand; two-one thousand; three-one thousand...up to ten." Then do the other arm/leg. You may find one side easier than the other. That probably shows that your hip muscle is stronger on one side than the other.

The plank

The plank is one exercise that can transform your core muscles and improve the way you hold your torso. I sometimes tell myself when standing or walking to get in 'plank position'. Immediately I stand taller and pull my navel back toward my middle back spine, a yoga strategy.

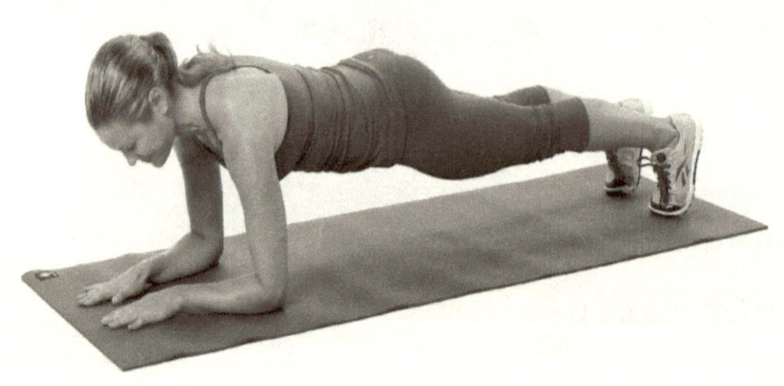

Begin by facing down with your weight supported by your elbows and toes. Your elbows should be directly under your shoulder. Keep your legs straight with your rib cage elevated. Now pull your navel back toward your spine. Be sure to keep your bottom tucked under.

Now count "one-one thousand, two-one thousand, three-one thousand" up to 30 this time! Increase your hold time to one minute as your core gets stronger.

There are numerous variations on the plank you can begin after you master the basic move. Just Google *Plank Variations*. Your abdominal muscles and back will thank you.

The dead lift

The dead lift trains my body to put all my energy in my hips. I still smile when I remember my brother, Dr. John, telling me if I wanted better balance, I had to get a stronger butt.

If you don't use your hip muscles to come back to standing while doing a dead lift, you run the risk of losing your balance. Trust me. I know.

Start standing tall holding a weight in each hand on the front of your thighs, just above your knees. With legs straight, bend at your hips without rounding your back. Run the weight down your leg until touching the floor. Then tighten your bottom to explosively come back to standing. Remember to use only the muscles in your booty and not just momentum. When you bend at the hip think "bottom out." When you come back up to standing think "bottom under."

I always heard to bend your knees when lifting something heavy to protect your back. Do that! Work your derriere, though, by contracting it to pull up to a straight leg stance. Try not to hyperextend your knees, but keep them slightly bent.

Start with light weights until you're certain you're really activating your hip muscles. Then you can increase the weight. Perform 10-12 repetitions.

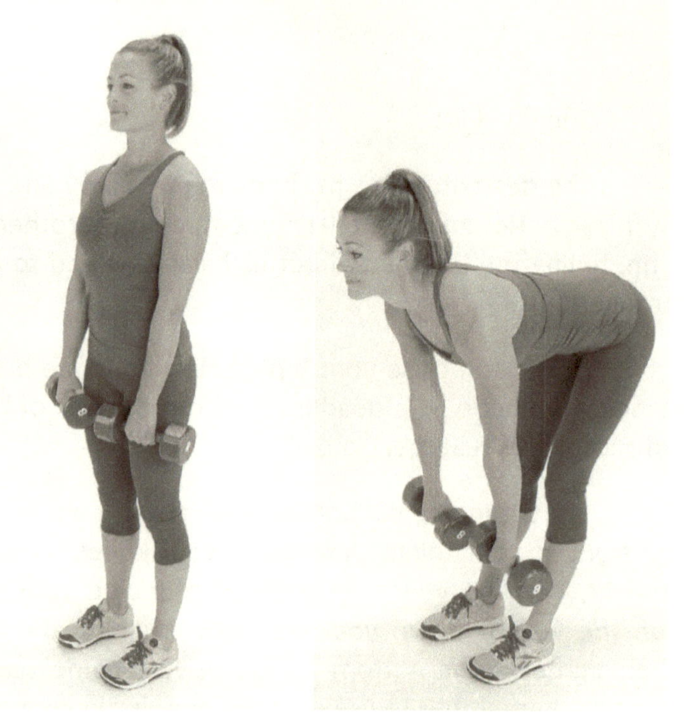

Chapter 17

The Diabetes Challenge

*To this end I strenuously contend with all
the energy Christ so powerfully works in me.*

Colossians 1:29

I love food, always have! Being a petite person made it easy for what I ate to end up on my hips and thighs. Unfortunately, I've had the appetite of an active man. So I quickly learned how to eat low-calorie foods so I could eat a lot of them.

I had a general idea of what foods were good for me, but was mainly interested in their calorie count. When I began running I knew that carbohydrates were quick energy. It seemed practical for me to become a carbohydrate junkie. I knew that whole grains were better for you than white breads and pastas. That was the extent of my nutritional knowledge, though.

I can't run anymore, but seem to keep myself in perpetual motion between teaching exercise class and working out. I definitely need some tips on maintaining my energy balance. I've never had to manage a health condition like diabetes, but the guidelines recommended for them are a good health choice for all of us.

My guest author in this chapter, Mary Gaskins, is a Registered Dietitian and Certified Diabetes Educator. I've always known her either as Mary from Bible study; or Mary from Louisville Christian Writers. I guess we all wear multiple hats in this life. Mary was very helpful as I wrote my first book, *The Light Through My Tunnel*. Then it dawned on me that Mary would be a great guest author using her diet and nutrition background.

Let's read what Mary shares with us about maintaining an energy balance with what we eat, using diabetes as the affliction.

by Mary Gaskins, RDN, CDE

"I didn't study nutrition or nursing or health education," Debbie told me. "I was diagnosed with diabetes and have to learn those things, whether I like it or not!" Debbie's pancreas had stopped producing insulin, a hormone that facilitates the conversion of food to energy.

As a nutritionist, it is my privilege to help clients balance their food intake to provide the energy and nutrients required to keep bodies and minds strong and healthy. Normally, through the marvel of digestion: carbohydrate, protein, fat, and other nutrients we've consumed are identified and sent through the bloodstream to appropriate cells. This process is a symphony of hormones, enzymes and other cofactors working together to provide the balance required for essential functions of life. Everything is absorbed properly, our cells produce the energy we need, and excess is stored as fat to be used later.

When something in this system goes awry, we have an opportunity to study and research exactly how our amazing bodies work. Such is the case with diabetes, which has been studied for hundreds of years. Two types were eventually identified. In both, the problem is that sugar can't be absorbed from the bloodstream—but for different reasons. In type 1, the pancreas stops producing insulin, a hormone that makes it possible for body cells to absorb sugar. In type 2, the pancreas still produces insulin but the body's cells do not respond to it correctly. Both types of diabetes result in the amount of sugar in the bloodstream growing dangerously high, leading to severe health complications. (In recent years, more regulating factors are being discovered and researched.)

Diabetes is a condition affecting more than 30 million (United States) Americans. It's estimated that

90-95% have type 2, and around 5% have type 1. Chances are you know several people with diabetes.

Eating well and staying active play vital roles in managing diabetes. Weight gain can cause insulin resistance and increase risk for heart disease and high blood pressure. Keeping records of daily blood sugar testing, food intake, exercise, and medication is recommended. With insulin pumps and blood sugar sensors, data can also be uploaded online for easier monitoring.

People with diabetes find themselves in the position of having to act as their own healers. They have to take the medical and nutritional advice they are given and figure out how to put it into practice in their own lives. It isn't easy. And it's not an option.

Mary Tyler Moore, an actress who managed type 1 diabetes throughout her career, was Debbie's role model.

"I think the best diabetes educators are the ones who have diabetes themselves!" Debbie informed me. I had to laugh and agree with her, even though that left me out of an elite group.

Studying nutrition and diabetes qualifies me to teach some basic principles, but I have always learned the most from my co-workers with diabetes, and diabetes support groups.

There's something about sharing with others that gives us strength. Our best support groups are made up of a mix of individuals who have managed diabetes for years, those who are newly diagnosed, and people with different types of diabetes.

If (as in type 1 diabetes) a person's body stops producing insulin, it must be taken by injection to enter the bloodstream. Insulin regimens vary according to individuals, and dosages are adjusted regularly depending on activity, medical conditions, changes in food intake, and even stress conditions. Persons with type 2 diabetes may be able to manage their blood sugar levels through diet and exercise; they may need medication to help their pancreas boost production of insulin, or to help their cells respond better to the insulin they do make. Sometimes insulin is prescribed for a person with type 2 diabetes. Some people have diabetes that does not fit neatly into a type 1 or type 2 category.

Support groups are a good way to learn how complicated managing diabetes can be. Those who have had diabetes longest are the ones least likely to criticize. Their sharing is often simple: "This is what works for me."

***

Here's a peek inside a support group:

Dave: "Why do I have to 'self-manage' my diabetes? I'm a truck driver. How can I eat a balanced diet and exercise on the road?"

Suggestions ranged from packing a cooler with sandwiches, fruit and vegetables, to bringing favorite menus from restaurants to the next meeting to determine the best food choices. An occupational therapist was scheduled to give the group advice regarding exercise on the job.

Jennifer: "This should not have happened to my daughter—she's done everything right! Food, exercise, she's been perfectly healthy! Why would her pancreas suddenly stop making insulin?"

Jennifer's daughter was 9 years old, slender, and a soccer player. There was no answer to Jennifer's question. Since the cause of type 1 diabetes is unknown, the conversation turned to advocacy for research. We were reminded that insulin was discovered around 100 years ago. The Nobel Prize for its discovery was awarded in 1923. Treatment and life expectancy for people with diabetes has improved dramatically, and there is still much to learn.

Molly: "The kids at school think diabetes is catching. They won't believe that I'm okay. My teacher doesn't understand why I need something sweet when my blood sugar drops."

The diabetes educator offered to call Molly's school and encourage the school nurse to talk with the teachers and class. Molly was also given information on diabetes summer camps for children. (diabetescamps.org)

Sarah: "Everyone wants to give advice on what I should eat. 'If you would just eat my way, you wouldn't have diabetes anymore.' Holidays are difficult. It ranges from: 'Here, just a little bite won't hurt you,' to 'Why are you eating that? Are you trying to make your diabetes worse?'"

Sarah had type 2 diabetes and had lost 30 pounds in the past year. She could maintain her blood sugar in a normal range if she stayed on the meal plan she had designed with the dietitian, but it was difficult. The group helped her work out a party strategy so she wouldn't arrive hungry, and could counter unwanted advice graciously. It helped to hear that everyone in the support group experienced similar situations.

Christy: "I have gestational diabetes. It's not type 1 or type 2, and it will last until my baby's born. I'm in my second trimester and I might have to start insulin before the baby comes."

Christy was already checking her blood sugar four times a day and following her meal plan closely. Her main concern was for her baby. The group encouraged her with success stories, and Molly demonstrated an insulin injection for her.

Sherman: "I'm a chef with type 2 diabetes. I'm all about presentation of beautiful food. Now I'm thinking, 'How many carbs are in this?'"

Sherman's joy in food preparation was inspiring, and he contributed several ideas to keep Christy and Sarah from meal-planning burnout. The group reviewed a carbohydrate counting guide from Lilly Diabetes.

***

Debbie (my client introduced at the start of this chapter) went back to school and became an expert diabetes educator. Because she has real experience with managing the condition, she inspires her patients and colleagues with her passion.

Diabetes is a unique health challenge. When a function as basic as converting food to energy is compromised, it highlights just how important wholesome eating is for a balanced life. So important, governments issue guidelines for good nutrition and fitness to encourage citizens to stay healthy.

The USDA offers ChooseMyPlate.gov as a guide to balance food choices, and SuperTracker.usda.gov to help people determine calorie needs, plan diets, and track progress toward goals.

***

Here are some helpful websites:

American Academy of Nutrition and Dietetics

eatright.org

Information on: healthy eating, nutrition facts and food labels, nutrition supplements,   grocery shopping, recipes, meal and snack ideas.

American Diabetes Association

diabetes.org

Information on: diabetes diagnosis, types, prediabetes, risks, symptoms, food, recipes, fitness with diabetes, diabetes camps, diabetes expos, research, advocacy.

diabetes.org/diabetes-basics/gestational

Information on gestational diabetes

Lilly Diabetes

lillydiabetes.com/_assets/pdf/ld90766_carbguide. pdf

Information on carbohydrate counting

lillydiabetes.com/programs-resources.aspx#downloadable

Downloadable basic diabetes information

Diabetes Self Management

diabetesselfmanagement.com/nutrition-exercise/mealplanning/

cooking-with-herbs-and-spice

Information on nutrition and meal planning

Diabetes Education and Camping Association

diabetescamps.org

Diabetes camps for children

USDA

choosemyplate.gov

supertracker.usda.gov

***

You may also enjoy reading:

Growing Up Again: Life, Loves, and Oh Yeah, Diabetes by Mary Tyler Moore

Mary Tyler Moore

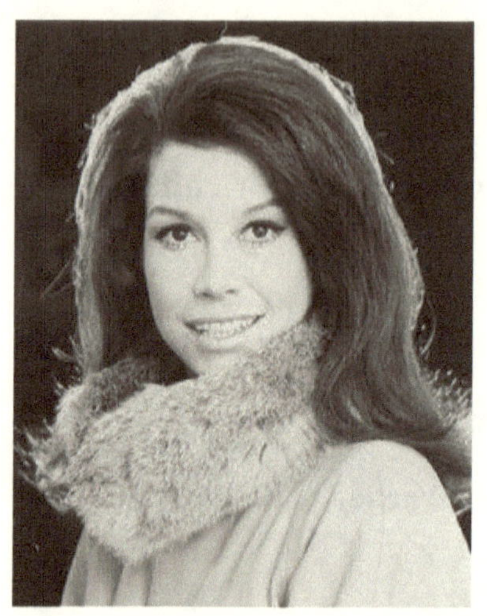

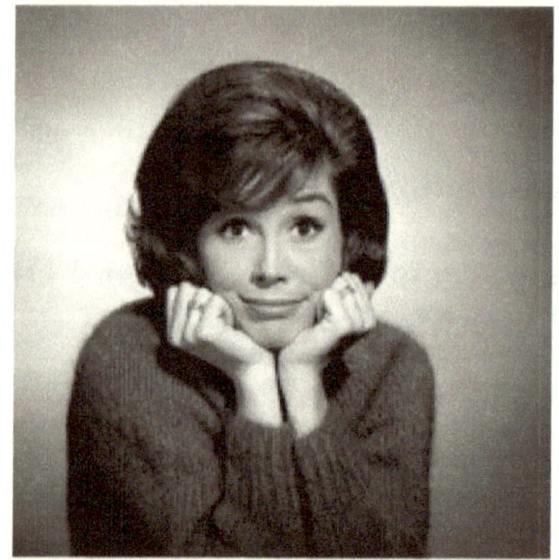

Chapter 18

The Mind

Love the Lord your God with all your heart and with all your soul and with all your mind and with all your strength.

Mark 12:30

We are tri-part beings; body, mind and spirit. Why is it the **mind** part that always trips us up? We feel uneasy. We feel unqualified. We had our mind set in another direction. We just don't want to put forth the effort. We're afraid.

Life is full of excuses, but if you don't think you can do something, you probably won't. The mind is powerful. Everything good and bad that happens will be processed in the mind with a verdict of either being a positive thing or a negative thing. Then we decide to act or not act; to make the time or put it off until later. And if it makes us afraid, all bets are off.

How we think will ultimately determine how we will live. How those around us think will make things even more challenging. My favorite Christian author/preacher, Joyce Meyer, is always proclaiming that *You are what you think about.*

Now read what a counselor and a life coach tell us about managing our mind in the next chapter.

Chapter 19

So What's Your Problem?

The mind governed by the flesh is death, but the mind governed by the Spirit is life and peace.

Romans 8:6

Several years after my traumatic brain injury, a Christian friend recommended a Christian counselor 'in training' that would see me at a very affordable price … free! I hadn't received any counseling after my brain injury or my divorce, so I was eager to see what words of wisdom a counselor would give me.

Phill was very approachable and easy to talk to. Since I had never seen a counselor before, I assumed that was a job prerequisite. Then he made an unusual request. Phill asked me to read the book of Ruth in the Bible.

Luckily, Ruth is the shortest book in the Bible. I have a whole chapter in *The Light Through My Tunnel* that speaks to the book of Ruth and the kinsman redeemer that becomes the hero of Ruth's story.

Phill was able to comfort me and give me a feeling of peace about this odd life that had literally just happened to me by means of my disabilities. He made me feel that I did indeed still have control simply by changing the way I thought about things. Of course we both believed that God was the ultimate master of what happened in my life.

Now read Phill's advice on overcoming all kinds of life problems.

by Phill Drake, MA, Pathfinder Life Coach and Recovery Guide

When people enter my office, after filling out the paperwork and praying for God to help us to identify, confront and turn from any "stinking thinking"... I will often ask them why they decided to see me. Whatever reason they share will be what counselors refer to as the "presenting problem."

No matter what people describe as the "problem," the fact is that what they THINK is the problem is seldom the REAL problem!

Let me explain. Clients will tell me that they have a problem with their marriage, or problems with an addiction, or depression problems, or anxiety problems, or health problems, or financial problems, problems at work, problems in the church, family problems, social-media problems, technology problems, legal problems ...

Problems, problems, PROBLEMS! But in reality, whatever their circumstances, the "problem" is not so much WHAT they are facing ... the real "problem" is the way they are dealing with ... (or NOT dealing with) ... whatever they have identified as "the problem."

The fact that <u>different people can react to the same circumstances in completely different ways</u> tells us that the experience itself is not the actual problem. It is the way the experience is <u>interpreted</u> and <u>processed</u> that turns any set of circumstances into a "problem"... or into a manageable "challenge" with a relatively easy solution.

For instance, imagine you are taking a college course with a difficult professor who is known to be very exacting and inflexible. Historically, half of his students fail the course, and most feel fortunate to even get a C from him. But you are an A student who plans to graduate *summa cum laude*! So, you study for the final exam with sincere diligence, while most of your classmates simply skim the textbook and spend the night partying—since they assume that they will probably fail the class anyway. After the final exam is completed, the professor announces that he has decided to give everyone in the class a "B." The classroom erupts into excited cheers. But, how do YOU react? Can you imagine the thoughts going through your mind? Would you be thinking something like:

"That's not fair!"

"I studied harder than they did, and they are getting the same grade!"

"Getting a B will ruin my 4.0 grade average!"

"Why did I even bother trying so hard?"

"I hate the professor and everyone in this stupid class!"

Do you see how this illustrates the point that the circumstances aren't the "problem"? Everyone in the class had the SAME circumstances, but only YOU saw the circumstances as a "problem."

It is NOT the difficulties that you are experiencing that are the problem. The truth is that the real "problem" is in your MIND and the way you interpret and process your circumstances. But what exactly is the mind, and how do we teach our minds to interpret and process our circumstances in a healthier way?

First of all, the mind is not the same as your brain. Now, this can be confusing since your mind actually resides in your brain, but just as you live in a house but you are not a HOUSE, the mind is NOT the brain, even though it lives there. The fact is that the brain is also the center of emotions (what many would call your "heart"), but few people would refer to the brain as your heart. It is sort of like two different people living in a house. The people and the house are all different, but all three interact with each other. In the same way, the brain (which is a physical part of our "body") houses and interacts with our heart and mind. Body, heart, and mind influence and are being influenced by one another. As Mary pointed out earlier, the key to success is to balance Body, Mind, and Spirit.

So your brain is the physical part of your body that houses your mind. The way the brain interacts with the mind is like the way a computer is both "hardware" and "software." If either the hardware (wires, circuits, fans, screens, etc.) or the software (programming, apps, etc.) are messed up, then the computer does not function properly. If the brain is damaged by illness, genetics, trauma, or chemicals (illegal drugs and alcohol) then the mind will be negatively impacted. On the other hand, just as a computer can have perfectly operating hardware and still be rendered useless by hacking the software with bad programming, malware, viruses, etc., in the same way a healthy brain can still house a troubled mind that is corrupted by bad "programming." To have a truly healthy mind, both the brain and the thoughts it processes must be healthy.

As a counselor I have worked with both the "hardware" and the "software" of a person's mental condition. If a client shows any signs of brain impairment, I encourage them to seek medical treatment before we work on the "software." Only after a brain is free from chemical imbalances, addictive substances, and other progressive hindrances will we be able to work on "re-programming" the corrupted "software." That is why it is vital to seek out a qualified counselor who has been trained to recognize problems that need medical attention. Remember, no matter how pure the software, it can't operate effectively in a computer with inadequate or damaged hardware. In the same way, the best counseling in the world will not help someone who needs antidepressants, mood-stabilizers, or detox from mind-altering chemicals!

Once we are sure that our brains are operating at their highest potential, then we can work on replacing the old faulty "programming" with new healthier thoughts and behaviors. It is here that understanding the relationship of the BODY, MIND, (heart) and SPIRIT is crucial, for each influences the other.

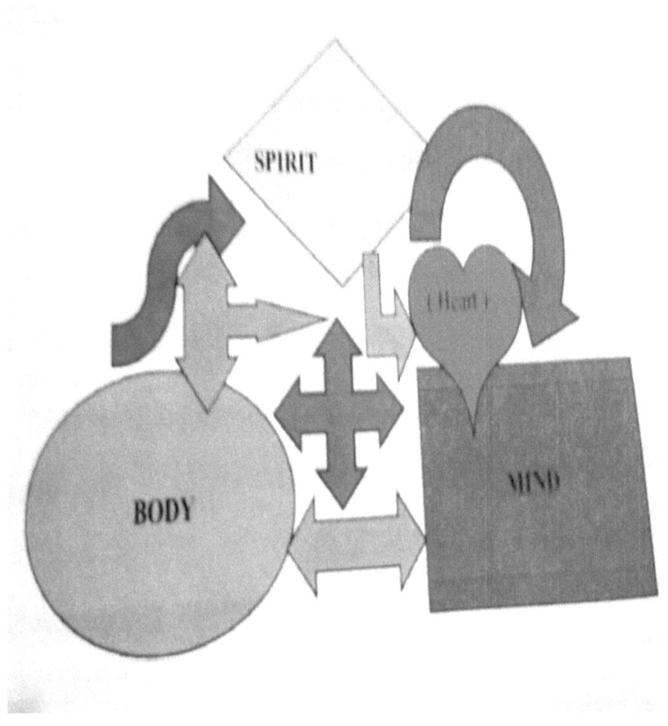

This dynamic interplay is discussed in various ways throughout the Bible, and sometimes terms like mind, soul, spirit, and heart are interchanged. As discussed earlier, the brain houses both the heart and the mind. Because they are so inter-related and influence each other, I will <u>consider them both part of the mind</u>. As such, to help distinguish them (although closely related) let us imagine them as a married couple—although <u>individuals with unique characteristics</u>, they are still <u>united as one</u>. The mind is the more rational, thoughtful, analytical spouse; and the heart is the more emotional, sensitive, and empathetic spouse. Balancing thoughts and feelings becomes vital for harmony in this heart/mind. That is why mental problems and emotional problems are so closely related and sometimes viewed the same.

Like most counselors, when helping clients work through their problems, I often ask them how they "feel" about a situation, because thoughts, feelings, and behaviors are so closely related. Sometimes they say they feel hopeless, discouraged, or unloved. Other times they say they feel angry, frustrated, or desperate. Regardless, in response I will often say something along the lines of:

"You FEEL what you feel, but the REASONS you feel might NOT be REAL!"

This goes back to recognizing that our "problem" is not so much our circumstances, but our interpretation and processing of the situations we experience. So when a wife says she doesn't feel loved because her husband is "always working" and "never" spends time with her, we discuss the meaning she has given to the situation and explore other possible explanations of his behavior. Often he will say something like:

"I wish I could spend more time with you, but I have to work to provide for you to show you how much I love you." Again, two vastly different emotional interpretations of the same set of circumstances. We then discuss how they each can understand and adapt to their different ways of expressing love to each other. This demonstrates the relationship between words, minds, and hearts.

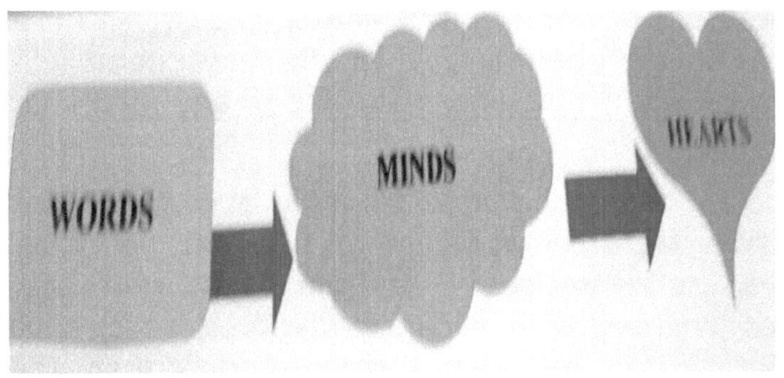

<u>Communications and experiences</u> are interpreted and formed into beliefs that generate emotions that motivate our behaviors.

Ideally the words are God's Truth that transforms our minds and purifies our hearts leading to proper actions. Unfortunately, they can also be lies that corrupt our minds and taint our emotions, leading to dysfunctional and sinful behaviors.

That is why the Apostle Paul said we need to offer our bodies (including our brains) as living sacrifices to God and stop conforming to the patterns (lies and sinful behaviors) of the world, but be transformed by the renewing of our minds (see Romans 12:1,2). He also instructs us to renew our minds by thinking about positive things instead of negative things (see Philippians 4:8). When we actively recognize, reflect, and redirect our negative thought patterns and the negative influences in our lives, then we can balance the interaction of body, mind, and spirit. Or, as I like to say in my opening prayer with my clients: "... identify, confront and turn from any "stinking thinking.""

For us to be able to truly accomplish the positive transformation of our mind, we must make sure we are seeing reality clearly. Years ago, I was counseling a recently-divorced recovering addict. When he enthusiastically described the mother of three he had met at the divorce-support group and detailed all the things he knew about her (including the fact that she worked at Hooters), I simply said:

"It's hard to see the red flags when you are looking through rose-colored glasses!"

After thinking about it for several seconds, he was able to laugh, and admit that his mind really wasn't processing information clearly. He realized that his heart and body (emotions and hormones) were overwhelming his mind at that point, so he needed to slow down and simply work on his recovery.

The above story illustrates how the mind can be fooled by the body. Another example of the body negatively impacting both the mind and the spirit is when health problems generate depression. Even allergies or the common cold (not to mention the flu) can make a person feel miserable. Think about it. Just how spiritual or mentally alert do you feel when you're sick? That is why it is so important to take care of our bodies with proper nutrition, exercise and adequate sleep. But many individuals suffer from chronic illnesses, or physical disabilities, or long-term mental health issues. Without proper treatment, these problems can overwhelm the mind and the spirit.

On the other hand, the mind itself can harm both the body and spirit. Our mind is where pride and selfishness and every sinful decision originates. The Bible says that the mind without the Spirit is hostile toward God, and cannot please him (see Romans 8: 5-7). A mind that ignores the Spirit makes all kinds of self-destructive decisions that harm the body, mind, and spirit (see Galatians 5:16-23). Every addict that comes into my office got there by following their "stinking-thinking" instead of following the Spirit!

This all goes to say that we must use our God-given minds to see clearly how important it is to take care of our bodies, minds, and spirits. All three were made to work together and to operate in harmony and balance. It is a valuable life-lesson learned when we manage to keep our body, mind, and spirit operating at the same speeds.

I can do all things through
Christ who strengthens me.

Philippians 4:13

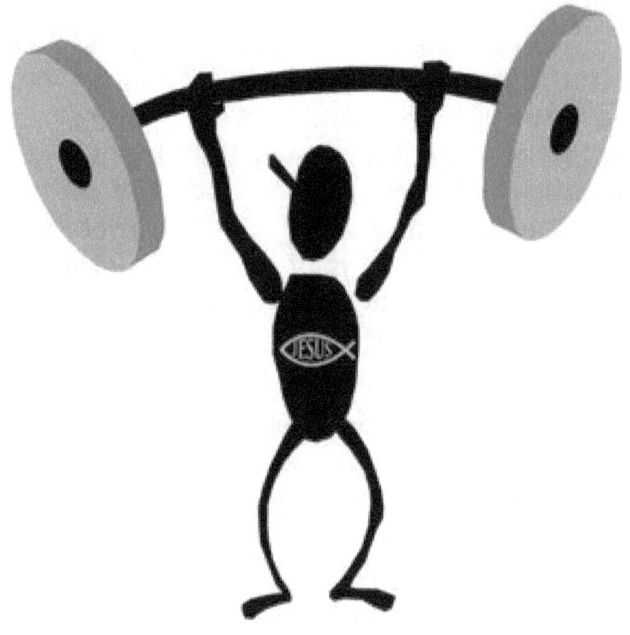

Chapter 20
Perspectives From a Life Coach

For the Spirit God gave us does not make us timid, but gives us power, love and self-discipline.

2 Timothy 1:7

I have spent so much time and effort in the last 20 years in trying to master and overcome my physical challenges that it took me almost 16 years to seek the advice of a counselor. I was so grateful just to be alive! Yes, my life had just changed drastically, but I thought all my woes would magically vanish if I became an able-bodied person again. I was certainly willing to work and wait for God's timing.

I met Elizabeth, the Life Coach, BEFORE she was a Life Coach. She was a recent widow who had started a social group called Singles Meeting Singles. I went to a couple of nice events feeling very awkward. I was disabled and moved about with great effort. My soft voice made it difficult to carry on a conversation in a noisy room. I felt invisible most of the time I was there, so I never went back. It was more comfortable being isolated at home.

Am I wrong to believe that God has a patient, loving man waiting for me? I've never felt comfortable in night clubs, but would go with girlfriends when I was younger. I met my ex-husband through a mutual friend. We both disliked the night life.

I'm older now, but still kind of cute. I discovered after my brain injury that it takes more than a pretty face to attract someone's attention. I'd like a man in my life again, but don't seem to be losing any sleep over it. Dating again sounds like a lot of work. What I really want is a family again. Can't I just skip the dating part?

I should continuously thank God for the opportunities he's placed in my life to impact others every day. I am blessed to have days filled with helping others by doing the very activity I love, which is exercising. Having a man in my life would change the way I do things. I'm a creature of habit and very content with my daily life. I am glad I now know a Life Coach, though, should I ever feel the need to modify my life and try something new. That has certainly happened before!

Now read these words of wisdom from Elizabeth. As a Life Coach, she gives us some useful tips to becoming more content with the life we have.

Hint: It has a lot to do with how we think.

Elizabeth Lewis, Life Coach

Our human brain is the most powerful muscle in our body. It's not actually a real muscle, but it behaves like one and controls all the other muscles; voluntary and involuntary. It is the most complex organ we have; made up of a complex network of billions of nerve cells called neurons. Everything we think and say, the way we move, the way we feel … all start in the brain.

The part we are going to uncover in this section has to do with the way we think. Isn't it amazing that we can have a thought and it can make us happy or sad? AND if we are having a sad thought, we can make our brain think of something happy and then feel happier? So, the question is, can we really control our way of thinking? I say YES!

Without getting technical, emotions happen when certain chemicals are present and those chemicals send messages to our body to feel a certain way (increased heart rate, higher blood pressure, and we might feel anger, pain, jealousy, happiness, etc.) This, then, can affect our mood.

Now, let's talk about what is holding YOU back. Each one of you is reading this for a glimmer of hope for your situation. You might be thinking, "Well, MY situation is different from anyone else's, so I'm sure you can't help me." Or "Maybe you have heard of this situation before. But you don't know me, so there is no way you (far away author who doesn't even know me) can help my personal situation." That is where you are wrong! The only thing holding you back from having a full life is you and your thinking … not your broken leg, your terminal diagnosis, your spouse cheating on you and your ugly divorce. Or even that you're overweight, you lost your job, you're in jail for embezzlement or you were raped and left for dead in a forest. (How awful if any of these things have happened to you.) My preacher once said, "These things are not happening TO you, they're happening FOR you." It just won't feel like it in the moment. There is opportunity in adversity. In fact, sometimes that is the one way out to a better place.

When something doesn't go our way (or if something doesn't meet our expectations), we tell ourselves a story. Brene Brown explained in a podcast interview that our brain is wired for survival, so we make up stories to protect ourselves. The story tells us who is good, who is bad, who is safe, etc. These stories need to be challenged because much of the time, the story we're telling ourselves isn't even true. But we go around trying to find evidence to prove our untrue story.

Here is an example. I work a lot with next-time-around singles. When they get back out there dating, they might have a few bad dates and start to wonder, "What is wrong with ME?" The story they make up is, "I'm not thin enough. Men like thin women. I'm not smart enough. Men like women who have been to college. I seem to attract all the wrong types of men. I must attract all the narcissists." Then the next time they have a bad date they'll say, "See? I told you I attract all the narcissistic men!" And the story isn't even true. They have just met men that have not met their expectations or that are not a good match. So they go through life with this untrue story in their head and feel less than normal.

Maybe your limitation is physical. You have 8 fingers and not 10. You're a little person, your skin has been burned or you have a club foot. Perhaps you think those limitations prevent you from finding love. Or finding the job you want. Or the friends you desire. We all formulate a belief system. I call it a limiting belief system. Many books have been written about this. Psychologists' offices are filled with people suffering in their heads and medication is given to those who find themselves in the darkest places mentally. I find this thinking to be a common thread with my life coaching clients.

So what do we do about this? How can we move forward?

First, recognize that these thoughts are going through your head. Examine them. Challenge them. In the coaching world, we call them our saboteurs. These are the voices in our head that tell us negative things about ourselves and we believe them to be true. The opposite of a saboteur is our sage (I call it your captain). It's that inner part of you that knows you like no other. The part of you that loves you, wants what is best for you, is full of wisdom and is positive because you're worthy. (If you were my client I'd walk you through a process to discover and recognize these parts of you more.)

Secondly, it's good to REFLECT. We all have to take ownership for our thinking and you need to ask yourself if what you're thinking is true. Is it really true? Every thought will either help you or hurt you. Ask yourself, "Does this thought help me or hurt me?"

This is an excerpt from the book, <u>Happiness is a Serious Problem</u>, by Dennis Prager. It's called The Missing Tile Syndrome. This definitely relates to our minds going to a negative place after something happens to us. "One of human nature's most effective ways of sabotaging happiness is to look at a beautiful scene and fixate on whatever is flawed or missing, no matter how small. This tendency is easily demonstrated. Imagine looking up at a tiled ceiling from which one tile is missing—you most likely concentrate on that missing tile. In fact, the more beautiful the ceiling, the more you are likely to concentrate on the missing tile and permit it to affect your enjoyment of the ceiling." This can be related to all of us because we always look at ourselves and see what is missing. We compare ourselves to others (and yes there will always be someone smarter, taller, thinner, prettier, more handsome, richer, etc). Comparison is definitely our worst enemy.

Back to what you can do about this. Every time you say a limiting belief, immediately turn it into a positive. Here are some examples:

Instead of saying…   Say….

"I'm never going to love again." → "Love is on the way to find me."

"No one will hire me because → "I have a lot to offer this company and I'm in a wheelchair … they are going to love me!"

"Because I had a stroke, I can't → "There is so much I STILL CAN do and I'm going to make a difference."

You get the idea. Write down all your limiting beliefs, and then turn each into a positive. There WILL be a positive. You just may have not thought of one yet. And heck … which one feels better? The positive one, right? Hire a Life Coach to walk you through this type of exercise, if needed. Put your hand over your heart. Feel that? If you feel your heart beating, YOU have PURPOSE. You just might need to reframe the way you think about it.

Affirmations

You may have heard about the power of positive thinking. I remember my father talking about this when I was growing up. Affirmations are similar to this, but more specifically, they are positive statements about yourself made in the present tense. This is an important aspect of the Law of Attraction (if you don't know about the Law of Attraction, look this up and learn about it). When reading this, you may think this is a silly practice. You may think this is only for women or for those with low self-esteem. While certainly helping low self-esteem folks, this is a good practice for us all: young and old, men and women. The purpose is to make you feel better, pour positive thoughts into your head, motivate and inspire you! They are always positive. You can repeat these affirmations whatever your circumstance.

If you don't repeat daily affirmations, why not start today? Write a few down. Say them in the present tense and say them until you believe them to be true! It's like studying for a test. You have to say the content over and over again in your head until you remember it. What can it hurt? No one else has to know you're saying them. I post these on my bathroom mirror and read them when I brush my teeth. They will make you feel good after saying them because they are true statements about the real YOU!

Our mind (and the thoughts we put in it) is a powerful tool. If we fill our brains with more negative than positive, then that's what we'll draw to us. Here are some examples of affirmations:

- I am beautiful/handsome.

- I am a strong, confident person.

- I have a good body.

- I am happy and full of joy.

- I am worthy and enough.

- God loves me and I love me.

- I'm successful and can handle anything that comes my way.

- My heart is open wide and I'm ready to love.

- Everywhere I go, I find love.

- Start today. Make a list of the top ten. Add to your list as needed. Start affirming the wonderful person you know you are.

Gratitude

You may have heard how important it is to live in a state of gratitude. I have heard this for years, and practiced this "when I remembered," but it wasn't until I watched *The Secret* and borrowed one of their ideas, that I actually started TRULY practicing gratitude every day! What do I do? I have a small rock/stone onto which I've typed/glued the word "gratitude." I put it in my pocket every morning, naming something for which I'm grateful. Throughout the day as I touch it, I name another thing for which I'm grateful; at day's end, yet another. When I began, I just named things for which everyone says s/he is thankful (kids, family, friends, house, food, job, etc.) But after a while I started naming things I would not say in a prayer to thank God for (i.e. dry underwear, multiple pairs of shoes, running water that can get hot or cold, clean pillow case, carpet under my feet). I always try to think of things I have not named before. This is how to truly live in daily gratitude. Then when things go wrong in life, I'm so used to being grateful that I see the blessings in the bad things that happen to me or my loved ones.

In August, 2015, I got an eye cancer diagnosis (uveal melanoma that was treatable), but I was told I would lose some eyesight after the first year. Even for someone like me who lived in daily gratitude, you wouldn't believe how blue the sky was (the same sky I saw and was grateful for the day before). How luscious the trees and flowers looked. The air smelled fresh, clean and crisp (even with the humidity). I saw more people smiling when I smiled at them. My skin felt softer. I saw the good in everyone even though they all were not always good. You get the idea. Even though I was not going to become totally blind, how grateful I was for all my senses (especially my eyes to see). All of a sudden all the petty things of the world fell away! Seriously, who cares if people make judgments, talk mean, if it rains when I want the sun to shine? Who cares if I'm cold with the A/C set on frigid; if my muscles hurt from working out; if my jeans are a little snug or my wrinkles are increasing in number? I am SO grateful for it all.

All this because I got a cancer diagnosis (and I will survive). How many people do you know that have been diagnosed with cancer? (I feel sure almost all of us can name several persons right now.) Or perhaps they have a different disease they didn't plan on having at an early age? I know there are so many with these diagnoses, partly because as I get older, my friends are also "aging" and new "diagnoses" are being discovered. Maybe your diagnosis is terminal and you only have a short time to live. Actually, we ALL only have a short time to live. Your situation is no different, really. The way you go might be different, but while you are here, you have a PURPOSE and your children and friends are observing how you deal with adversity. Maybe your purpose is to show them how to die? Gracefully. With love. Maybe your life will be extended due to your will to fight and live? Oh, how lucky we are with advanced technology, great doctors and more advanced treatments. So, when you look at your challenges, find a small rock or stone and start this habit of living in daily gratitude. It works and makes a difference. Then, you can share the idea with others.

"We cannot solve the world's problems at the same level at which they were created." -- Albert Einstein

The Spirit

What we have received is not the spirit of the world, but the Spirit who is from God, so that we may understand what God has freely given us.

1 Corinthians 2:12

The **Spirit** part of my being brings me the most comfort and is also a constant companion of mine. I suppose it's always been there; excuse me, I KNOW it's always been there, but it took a tragedy and a lot of loneliness before I finally recognized it (him). I've often heard that individuals find God most keenly in difficult times. As a believer, I already knew God's presence in my life. Like a child cries out for her parents, I instinctively cried out for God.

Through my affliction, my faith has grown tremendously. I've learned the power and peace that comes through prayer. Yet I keep reading, watching and praying for a closer walk with God. I suspect that need will continue until I'm finally home with him.

Now read what two individuals I consider to be spiritual giants say to us about finding a closer relationship with God ... even in afflictions.

Chapter 21

What Is God Telling You?

'Call to me and I will answer you and tell you great and unsearchable things you do not know.'

Jeremiah 33:3

After my accident and traumatic brain injury, I instinctively turned to God for comfort. Just like my parents, I knew he was always there. My accident happened in May 1997. I had not even heard of Bible study at that time, but my Catholic faith had given me a good sense of God's power in my life. I was begging, pleading and negotiating to get away from this mess my life had become.

I figured I had better get to know this Almighty Sovereign Lord a little better. I surely was going to be asking for his help. That is where my spiritual journey began. I became a voracious reader of Christian books, including books on healing. The healing books included numerous passages from God's word, the Bible. So I joined my first Bible study in Little Rock, Arkansas at the age of 38.

I was immediately impressed and intimidated by how well-versed these Christian women from other Protestant faiths were. As I said in my first book, they quoted scriptures like my brothers quoted sports scores. I sure did have a lot to learn!

My brain injury makes remembering new facts difficult, but meditation and memorizing have never been my strong suit. Just give me the basic facts and let me get it done. *"Be still, and know that I am God; I will be exalted among the nations, I will be exalted in the earth." Psalm 46:10 (NIV).* I'm trying, Lord! This is not natural for me.

I stayed with Bible studies not only to learn, but to be surrounded by others who believed as I do. My life became somewhat isolated when I became disabled, but you don't have to jump or run to be inspired by the Lord. Bible Study Fellowship (BSF) was the last Bible study I tried ten years ago. I've never left.

Our leader, Nancy, has so much passion for God's word. Even on the nights I'm not feeling inspired, I find myself listening and taking notes. I'm sure I will read and re-read the insights Nancy has given us here.

Nancy Ogle

Leader, BSF International

Life is hard and messy. It is confusing and full of expected and unexpected trouble and difficulty. Every one of us carries around with us burdens, woes, sorrows, and pain. Life is not easy. To be human is to know suffering. To be human is to experience heartache and disappointment. To be human is to feel pain. To be human is to desire answers, solutions, and explanations.

I believe that's why God gave us His Word, the Bible. When God looked at His creation and desired to give them help, He wrote a book. He supernaturally inspired men and women to write the 66 books that make up the Bible. God talks to us in the Bible. He speaks words of timeless wisdom and truth. He speaks words of unsurpassed encouragement and hope. He speaks words that are able to spark joy and delight.

My name is Nancy Ogle and I've taught the Bible in Bible Study Fellowship for over 24 years. When Mary asked me to be a contributor to her new book, I immediately said yes, because who can say no to Mary? She is a beautiful woman of God who lives her faith in ways that inspire all of us. So of course, I said yes!

Over my years of teaching, countless women have approached me for help. After lectures or through emails, phone calls or random encounters, women have shared their hurts and difficulties. They've told me about their heartaches and pain. I've heard stories that have left me in tears, crying out, "Jesus, come quickly."

One such story was Anna's. Anna was in a difficult marriage. Her husband was verbally abusive and showed no care or concern for her. He expected her to serve him, no questions asked. Anna's life was horribly difficult. The wonderful marriage she had hoped for had turned into a nightmare. She approached me one night after the lecture and we sat and talked. She tearfully told me what life was like for her on a daily basis. She had no hope and felt lost and alone. Her husband had no interest in God. He tolerated her attending Bible study, but she wasn't permitted to speak about it.

I listened. I prayed. There were many things I wanted to say to Anna that night. But what God wanted to say to her was more important. I wasn't who Anna needed. I didn't have answers and explanations. She needed to hear from God. She needed His words. She needed timeless truth and wisdom—unsurpassed hope— words that could spark joy in her heart even in her unimaginable pain. The help Anna needed couldn't be found in a human—it had to come from God.

I remember getting out my Bible and opening it to the passage we had studied that week. We looked at it together and I asked Anna what God had said to her. She said He had told her He loved her. We had been studying Romans chapter 8. I asked Anna to read Romans 8:37-39 and insert her name into the verses. Through tears she read and spoke aloud the truth of God's immense and real love for her.

We prayed and I invited her to come talk to me again. Anna's problems weren't solved that night. How could they be? But Anna left knowing a far greater reality than her broken marriage. Anna left with truth in her mind and heart. Timeless truths help us change the way we think about our problems. They fuel our resolve. They ignite hope and enable us to go on one more day. Hearing from God eased her hurt just a little.

I believe God designed us to need His Word. He designed us to require to hear Him speak into our lives. He created us with a mind to think. We are thinking beings designed by our Creator to use our mind to interact with God's Word and then use His words as an interpretive grid for all of life. The Bible is God's interpretive grid that enables us to not just function in times of difficulty, but to flourish.

The Bible gives us truth and wisdom, but most importantly, the Bible gives us God Himself. God reveals Himself in His Word and He is what we need most in this life. Turning to the Bible in times of trouble keeps us personally connected to God. When we turn to the Bible, we turn to God. He is there, eager to speak to us intimately. To read the Bible is to commune with God.

Her name was Joyce. We ran into each other in the cereal aisle of Kroger. She told me she was in our class and was really enjoying the study. I quickly realized she wanted to talk about something more important than just what cereal was on sale. Joyce explained that she had just learned that her breast cancer had returned and it didn't look hopeful. She had a husband and two teenage daughters. Life is hard.

We hugged and right there in the cereal aisle I prayed with her. She told me that God was flooding her with evidence of His care for her and her family. She said each day He spoke to her through her Bible reading. She told me His voice had never been louder or clearer. Joyce chose to stay close to God. She eagerly and expectantly read His Word each day, letting it wash over her and drench her with God's grace and mercy.

God's Word is our lifeline. It keeps us tethered to the One who gave us life and the One who sustains our life. As we open up the Bible God begins to speak, whispering His comfort, drenching us with His grace, shouting His promises, reminding us of His presence and flooding our mind and heart with truth and wisdom we desperately need. What we need most in times of difficulty is to hear from the One who loves us more than we could ever imagine. We need time with our Creator, the One who knows everything about us and our situations, relationships, desires and dreams. We need God to speak into our lives a greater reality than our pain, our trouble, our heartbreak, our confusion, our sorrow.

God reveals Himself in the Bible. Using human language, God makes Himself known. Using words any literate person can read, God speaks. He communicates with His creation. From the very beginning God is described as someone who speaks. God created the universe using words. God said, "Let there be light," and there was light. God spoke the universe and everything in it, into being. God's Word, His chosen way to create and communicate with His creation, is His identity. It cannot be separated from His essential nature and character.

When God created humanity, He created it with the capacity for language. God in His amazing grace desires to communicate with us, and so He created us with the ability to do so. God's language is the language of His creation. And just as human relationships depend on communication, so does our relationship with God. We speak to God through prayer. God speaks to us in the words of the Bible.

It's interesting and very telling to realize that the Bible says very little about seeing God, but it says volumes about hearing Him. We hear Him in the words of the Bible. The path to hearing God travels though the Bible—from words on a page into our minds and then into our hearts. Trace that path with me. We open the Bible. God speaks through the words on the page. His words enter our mind as we read and process what He is saying. His personal message to us travels from our mind to our heart. God has touched us with His truth.

God wants us to live life and handle life with other people. We should talk and listen to friends and family, pastors and counselors. These resources are all part of His faithful care and provision for us. But nothing and no one can replace hearing from God personally through His Word. Just ask Patricia.

Patricia sought me out one night just as I was leaving the church. She wanted to know if I had a few minutes to talk with her. I did. We sat in my car and I listened to her story. Her husband had recently died. He was killed in a car accident. Just like that her world changed. She was alone. She had lost her first love and best friend. Her grief drove her to God, she told me. She said that the only way she had survived was hearing Him speak words of comfort to her. She told me of sleeping with her Bible and using her cellphone's flashlight at night to read it when she woke up and couldn't get back to sleep. She told me of keeping a Bible in every room of the house opened to passages and verses that spoke of God's love, God's nearness, God's comfort. She told me of listening to her audio Bible in the car. She said saturating herself with God's Word like this kept her focused and thinking right. It kept her focused on the greater reality—God's real presence—God's real power—God's real love.

We need God's Word to speak into our pain. We need to hear God tell us what to do, what to think, what to focus on, what matters most. Without God's word we are left to navigate life in our own understanding of things. Without hearing from God, we listen too closely to ourselves, to others and to this world. Without God speaking truth into our lives, we will believe lies. Without God's message to us our lives won't make any sense.

We need to hear God speak to us because we are human beings. We are weak, frail, sinful, broken, and messy people—living in a broken and messy world. We have no means to understand and make sense of this world and our lives apart from divine help. God knew that, so He wrote a book. He created language and uses language to speak to His creation. I am utterly amazed by that. I hope you are, too.

I have learned in my own personal life that this world distracts, that my flesh is weak and that Satan is active. These real hindrances keep me from hearing God speak. My personal life can get crazy busy. This world constantly tempts me to waste my time. Satan works to fill my mind with lies. So hearing from God, reading His Word, saturating myself with His message to me, must be an intentional decision each day. It's the only way it's going to happen.

The Bible, God's Word, puts me in touch with God's thoughts about me and my life and this world and others. It connects me to what God wants to tell me about everything in this world and in my life. I need to hear that daily. I can't hear that enough. And neither can you.

Life is hard and messy. It is confusing and full of expected and unexpected trouble and difficulty. On good days and bad God has a word of truth for us. On good days and bad there are things God wants to tell us, remind us of, open our hearts to, convict us of and more. I can't begin to even list everything God wants to tell you and me. All I know is that He does.

That's why God has created us in His image with minds that can understand and process language. That's why He wrote a book and included in it a personal message of truth for us. Many things can be said about the Bible—but perhaps the most important thing that can be said about it is this: In it we hear the very words of God Himself. His words give life. His words offer real hope. His words soothe and comfort. His words answer life's hardest questions. His words lead to freedom. His words defeat sin. His words lead to lasting joy. His words were written for you.

People often ask me questions like, "How long should I read the Bible each day?" "What should I read?" "Where should I start?" I always begin answering these questions by saying, "There is no magic formula or plan." And there isn't. The Bible is unlike any other book. Every word, every verse, every passage is of infinite worth. How can you even begin to suggest guidelines for reading it? Yet, because we are who we are as people, we do need some practical help. Here are three tips for reading the Bible, for hearing God speak to you and into your life.

1. Make the decision to read from the Bible every day. There are hundreds of Bible-reading plans on the Internet. Just google *Bible Reading Plans* and you'll find plenty to choose from. Choose one that fits best with the amount of time you can give each day. Most importantly—just determine to do it. Determine each day to hear a word from God!
2. Read your Bible with a pen ready to underline, mark and make notes either directly on the pages of the Bible or in a notebook. Just as you might take notes when a person is speaking to you so you don't forget what they've said, you'll want to do the same thing as God speaks to you each day!

3. Pray before and after you start. Ask God to speak truth, encouragement, help, conviction into to your current situations, relationships, trials and difficulties. Ask Him to open your heart and mind to hear from Him and receive His words with a willingness to listen and obey. When you finish return to Him in prayer expressing thanks and asking for His help and power to enable you to be changed, inspired, moved by the words He has just spoken to you.

Reading the Bible is hearing from God Himself. The Bible is the very word of God. God, who spoke face-to-face with Moses as a man talks to his friend, still speaks to people today, people like you and me. God speaks. When you open the Bible God is not distant, He is near. When you read the Bible, God is not silent, He is talking to you. The Bible you hold in your hands, written in a language you can understand, is the Word of God. It is exactly what God determined to say to you and me. May we listen well. May we listen and be quieted by His voice, comforted by His truth, encouraged by His actions, moved by His power, amazed by His goodness, humbled by His greatness, changed by His grace, and forever overwhelmed by His love.

I can do all things through
Christ who strengthens me

Philippians 4:13

Chapter 22

Rejoice In Hope

Love must be sincere. Hate what is evil; cling to what is good. Be devoted to one another in love. Honor one another above yourselves.

Romans 12:9-10

Father Shayne is our new, young pastor at St. Raphael the Archangel Catholic parish. He's like a breath of fresh air! One of the first changes I noticed after his arrival is that he started ringing chimes again during the Eucharistic celebration at Mass. That's a ritual that had fallen away from the Mass in recent years.

Ringing the chimes draws your attention to the altar, where the bread and wine are being transformed by the touch of the priest's hands into the body and blood of Christ. It immediately brought back memories of my mother bowing her head and tapping her chest as the chimes rang.

I know there are numerous Christian denominations and that God loves every one of us. The Catholic faith is my lifelong religion that places a special emphasis on the Eucharist when the bread and wine actually become Jesus's body and blood. So I'm all for the chimes being back!

Father Shayne is a wonderful preacher. We call his message the *homily* in the Catholic Mass. The homily usually references one or all of the three scripture readings from that Mass. Many times it feels like Father Shayne is speaking directly to my heart. It's the same way I feel like God is speaking to me sometimes when I hear the message from a minister on television.

Now read what Father Shayne has to say about the qualities of Rejoicing, Enduring and Persevering.

Rejoice in Hope, Endure in Affliction, Persevere in Prayer

Romans 12: 12

I have found this passage from Sacred Scripture to be very challenging and important to me. I am sure I have heard this passage many times before and just ignored it. I fell in love with it and it resonated with me in a profound way while I was in seminary at Saint Meinrad Seminary and School of Theology in Saint Meinrad, Indiana. We were preparing to celebrate the season of Lent and the formation team felt like St. Paul's letter to

the Romans would be of a particular interest to us as we prepared to journey through the season of prayer, fasting, and almsgiving. Now, as a priest and pastor, but more importantly, as a man—a child of God, created in His likeness and His image, I am even more passionate about this particular passage because it contains a simple yet attainable roadmap on how to live our life.

Some of us are proud of our faith, our denominations, our religion. Others have fallen away from actively practicing their faith, while others seem to claim to be spiritual but not religious. If we listen to what St. Paul tells us in these nine simple words, then our lives could ultimately be changed for the better. I know they have gotten me through some pretty rough times.

When Mary asked me to write a chapter for her book from the spiritual perspective, I was a little unsure about being able to do it. I do not consider myself to be an avid reader of books, nor do I consider myself to be a writer. Mary calmed my fears by simply asking me to write as if I was preparing to deliver a sermon. Now that I can do! I love to preach the Word of God; preparing for sermons/homilies gives me great joy and excitement because I truly do believe people want to hear the Word of God. People are craving to hear the truth—the genuine truth that will ultimately set us free. Freedom from pain and suffering, freedom from the burdens of sin and temptation, and freedom from being possessed by the very things we think bring us great joy, when in fact they only cause us emptiness and loneliness. Nothing is better than leaving Mass or church services with a powerful, yet simple message—a message of hope, endurance, and perseverance.

In this chapter, I will attempt to share with you reasons to be hopeful. I will help you understand why sometimes we just have to endure the pain and the suffering that we are dealt and endure it as best we can. Thirdly, I will share with you the need to pray … to pray always, no matter what the reason might be, no matter if it is a prayer of thanksgiving, or a prayer of deep demands and desires.

I am a 35-year-old Roman Catholic priest. I have been ordained only 3 years, and I am currently the pastor of a large parish in Louisville, Kentucky. I am a young, inexperienced, passionate person, who loves and cares for the sheep entrusted to my care. As a pastor, I am their shepherd and I have the responsibility of making sure they are cared for, protected, and most importantly saved, so that one day, at a time none of us knows, we will see our Lord and Savior in the Eternal Banquet of Heaven. Mary Varga is one of my parishioners and she inspires me on a daily basis. When I see and interact with Mary, I see the pain and the suffering that she has endured, but I also see a smile on her face, always a smile, and she, like so many others, gives me great hope and comfort in knowing that life should not be taken so seriously and that we need to live life to the fullest. Life is precious, life is sacred, and it can be taken away from us in an instant.

Rejoice in Hope

What does it mean to rejoice? What does it mean to hope? When I hear the word rejoice I often think back on memories. I think back to happier times when I was a child, not a care or worry in the world. These memories are precious and they help tell a story. We all have them. Some are good memories, while others are sad and painful. I love looking at old photographs of family and friends; black-and-white photos of people who appeared to be living in simpler times. They were smiling and laughing, they were engaged with one another, and it appeared as though no one was glued to a particular electronic device that took up most of their time and energy. These memories—these people from the past— were creating opportunities to rejoice. As a priest I am always looking for ways to promote and share the Good News with others. When I think of rejoicing, I think about the good news that needs to be shared. Have you ever heard or received such good news that you were bursting at the seams and excited to share it with someone else? Perhaps it was your first job, your first kiss, your acceptance into a particular school. Perhaps you finally made the sports team you worked so hard to be a part of. Maybe this need to rejoice came at a time when you were about to give up. You had exhausted all your resources, you had nowhere to turn, and all it took was this good news, this exciting opportunity to give you a new outlook on life. As a pastor, people often come to me for guidance and advice. They are looking for reasons to rejoice, especially when there is nothing in their life that warrants any reason to hope. That is when I recall memories. Remember what it felt like to be loved? Remember what it felt like to get that good news? Remember the trials, the pain, the suffering, and hard work you put into a particular cause or situation that gave you reasons to hope? I often think of a couple who is having the most difficult time conceiving. They sit in church every weekend only to see other couples their age having children, getting them baptized, getting them registered for school, and as much as the couple struggling to conceive wants to be happy for them, they are most likely miserable on the inside. And then their prayers are answered, they are finally pregnant, and they rejoice. They rejoice because now they have a reason to be hopeful.

I think we must ask the question: are we optimistic about life, or are we pessimistic? Do we first see the good in others or are we constantly searching for the bad? Do we trust one another so that we can share our joys, our trials, and our experiences with them? Do we find opportunities every day to simply rejoice—to laugh, to smile, to love, and to forgive? Hope is powerful, especially when we stop to give thanks for reasons to hope. A person of hope can take the good with the bad. They can see that this trial or this struggle will soon pass and something good or better is right around the corner. A person who lacks hope will tend to be a miserable person. What is there to be excited about? What is there to look forward to? Why do I need to engage with others? Why do I need to care? Because that is why we were created. God created us in His image and likeness, and God does not make mistakes. Just look at the beauty of creation. The sunrises, the sunsets, the changing of the colors of the leaves, the warm sun, the cool winter breeze. Each day is an opportunity for us to be a person of hope, a person who rejoices in the cards that we are dealt; whether they are good or bad, they are ours and they show us that rejoicing in hope will pave the way for an attitude of joy, love, happiness, and excitement. My friends, rejoice and be glad and then share that good news with others.

Endure in Affliction

Pain is inevitable. Even the most optimistic, carefree, joyful person will experience immense pain and suffering. Now, how a person deals with pain and suffering makes all the difference in the world. As a pastor, I see pain and suffering on a daily basis. I first see it when I look into the mirror every morning. I am a happy person, who appreciates life, and is thankful that God called me to the vocation of priesthood. But not every day is happy, joy-filled, or awesome. I am reminded of my pain and brokenness on a daily basis. Being a priest and a public person is hard. People expect many things of us. They expect us to be at five different places all at the same time. They expect us to drop what we are doing and attend to their particular needs or wants, and for the most part we do just that. We drop what we are doing to help minister to the needs of others, to be with them in their time of need, their time of trial and despair. And when certain expectations are not met people lose hope in us and in the Church. They become angry, hurt, and resentful. I have had those same feelings throughout my life and my ministry.

What does it mean to endure something? People will often tell me that they are not really sure how much more they can handle. One more hurtful or painful experience will push them over the edge. I try my best to counsel them, because I have been there myself, to sit with the pain, to sit with the suffering, and place themselves at the foot of the cross. Now, look up! What do you see? You hopefully see Christ looking down at you. As drops of blood and sweat fall from his face, you see a man who was beaten and torn up, a man who was put to death to set each and every one of us free. You see a man who loves us so much that he died for us. In order to have the resurrection you first had to have the crucifixion. When we are experiencing pain, sadness, depression, and despair, we have to trust that the pain will either pass or subside and that a new opportunity is on the horizon. Suffering happens to people who are rich and who are poor. Suffering happens to people who are public figures and hidden ones too. Suffering has no bias toward sex, age, or race. We cannot avoid it. It is what we do with suffering that makes all the difference in the world, especially if we strive to be people of hope. Enduring affliction is very painful, and we cannot do it alone. God did not create us to be alone, He created us to be in communion with one another. Don't try and fight these battles, these sufferings alone. Talk to someone who has been there before. Be open, be honest, be vulnerable and let others help you. I have always struggled with that. I think that I can solve all my problems by myself. I don't want to burden anyone else with my problems, and then I quickly realize that people want to be helpful, people actually do care, and they want to make sure they can help in any way possible. Let them help you. Let them help carry whatever crosses you bear, either daily ones, or those that are just for a moment. Remember, sometimes we have to experience pain, loss, suffering, and afflictions, in order to be changed for the better. Hope allows us to see that something greater is happening and that we will be okay, as long as we take it one day at a time. One of the greatest ways we can get through these difficult times is to take it all to God in prayer—to speak to God about our joys and our sufferings, and to let Him help us get through it all.

Persevere in Prayer

I hope you have reasons to hope. I hope you have found ways to endure affliction. But have you been able to persevere in prayer? What does it mean to pray? Just because I am an ordained priest of Jesus Christ, does not mean I have a direct phone line to the Man upstairs. Every single day, people will call me, text me, email me, or stop me and ask me to pray for them or for someone else. I am sure this has happened to you, especially if family or friends know you practice your faith and that you do believe in answered prayers. We help make up the Communion of Saints here on earth. All of our prayers are heard, but perhaps not as immediately as we hope. We are striving for greatness, we are striving to make a difference, and we are hopeful that the prayers we share will be heard and answered. But when our prayers are not answered when we want them to be answered, we must not give up, we must persevere in our prayers. God hears us, there is no doubt about that, but we must trust that our prayers will be answered according to His will and in His time. When you pray, you have to ask yourself this simple question: Are you doing most of the talking or are you listening? Prayer is simply a conversation with God. It is a dialogue. And like any dialogue there have to be two parts, speaking and listening. Healthy dialogue requires a good balance of both.

Often when people say they are tired of praying, or they are talking to God but not getting any immediate results, odds are they are not taking the time to listen. When we are able to persevere in our prayers, we are able to go to that quiet place in the depths of our souls and actually listen to Jesus speaking to us. Even the greatest saints of the Church experienced dryness in their prayers. They begged, they pleaded, they fought, they listened to God, and sometimes their prayers were answered and sometimes they were not. In order for us to speak to God we have to go to the depths of our souls. We have to have the patience and the perseverance to trust, to listen, and to respond. I have a good spiritual director and he is always challenging me to seek God in all that I say and do. He often asks me, 'Where is God in this particular situation?' Sometimes I can see God clearly, other times, not so much. I also want to be the best priest and pastor that I can be, but he recently challenged me to strive to be a better man first; then strive to be a better Christian, then persevere to be a better priest. I think this is true for all of us no matter what our vocation or life status may be. We must all strive to be better, to be that better person God has created us to be. Then we can be a better spouse, a better friend, a better son or daughter. We can be a more joyful person, we can endure any affliction God gives us, and our prayer life and our perseverance in that prayer will only deepen, knowing that through it all, through all the ups and downs in life, we can say without hesitation that our life has meaning and that our life has a purpose.

My dear brothers and sisters, through it all, always remember to Rejoice in Hope, Endure in Affliction, and Persevere in Prayer.

EPILOGUE

Closing remarks by Mary Varga

***

Not only so, but we also glory in our sufferings, because we know that suffering produces perseverance; perseverance, character; and character, hope. And hope does not put us to shame, because God's love has been poured out into our hearts through the Holy Spirit, who has been given to us.

Romans 5:3-5

***

In the above Bible passage, the word *suffering* can be substituted with the word *affliction*. We all live with them. Afflictions can be small or great. They can be temporary or life-long. What makes the ultimate difference for a contented and peaceful life is how we deal with them.

I am not a doctor, a therapist or a counselor. I am simply sharing with you tips that have enabled my body; enlightened my mind; or recharged my spirit. I am a certified personal trainer who knows how best to work with my body. I have a tendency to push myself too hard physically. That is why I rely on other experts to help me map out a game plan.

I've attempted to show you many ideas for managing the troubles/afflictions you may face in your life. It's certainly not going to solve all your problems, but just knowing you're not the only one struggling can make the battle a little less overwhelming. Right? We are never alone in this journey of life.

Hold tight to the recommendations relating to the mind and spirit. Just like our bodies need continual training to be their best, we need to continually monitor what we allow to come into our minds, then trust God to hold it all together for us.

Working with my many guest authors has given me a magnificent feeling of fellowship and camaraderie. It also confirms for me that people truly do want to help. They have put their heart and soul into their writing … and they did it for you.

Please keep this book nearby so you can refer back to the suggestions and information it contains. Reading a book for enjoyment is one thing. My hope is that you will refer back to *The Afflicted Healer* for facts or maybe inspiration to keep you going. May the information contained in this book move you closer to the active, peaceful life of purpose you deserve!

Scripture Appendix

I began each chapter of this book with a Bible verse relating to the subject being discussed. Below you will find many scriptures that could also have been used.

I've divided them into: BODY, MIND, SPIRIT, and AFFLICTIONS/SUFFERING. I'll be looking to these for encouragement and inspiration.

<u>Body</u>

<u>Mark 2:17</u>

On hearing this, Jesus said to them, "It is not the healthy who need a doctor, but the sick. I have not come to call the righteous, but sinners."

Proverbs 4:13

Hold on to instruction, do not let it go; guard it well, for it is your life.

Matthew 6:22

The eye is the lamp of the body. If your eyes are healthy, your whole body will be full of light.

1 Corinthians 6:19-20

Do you not know that your bodies are **temple**s of the Holy Spirit, who **is** in you, whom you have received from God? You **are** not your own; you were bought **at a** price. Therefore honor God with your bodies.

John 2:21

But the **temple** he had spoken of was his body.

2 Corinthians 5:10

For we must all appear before the judgment seat of Christ, so that each **of** us may receive what is due us for the things done while in the body, whether good or bad.

Galatians 2:20

I have been crucified with Christ and I no longer live, but Christ lives in me. The life I now live in the body, I live by faith in the Son of God, who loved me and gave himself for me.

1 Thessalonians 5:23

May God himself, the God **of** peace, sanctify you through and through. May your whole spirit, soul and **body** be kept blameless at the coming **of** our Lord Jesus Christ.

1 Corinthians 12:12-27

Just as a **body**, though one, has many parts, but all its many parts form one **body**, so it is with Christ. For we were all baptized by one Spirit so as to form one **body**— whether Jews or Gentiles, slave or free—and we were all given the one Spirit to drink.

Matthew 5:29

If your right eye causes you to stumble, gouge it out and throw it away. It is better for you to lose one part of your **body** than for your whole **body** to be thrown into hell.

Matthew 6:22

The eye is the lamp of the **body**. If your eyes are healthy, your whole **body** will be full of light.

Matthew 6:25

Therefore I tell you, do not worry about your life, what you will eat or drink; or about your **body**, what you will wear. Is not life more than food, and the **body** more than clothes?

Luke 11:36

Therefore, if your whole **body** is full of light, and no part of it dark, it will be just as full of light as when a lamp shines its light on you."

Mark 14:22

While they were eating, Jesus took bread, and when he had given thanks, he broke it and gave it to his disciples, saying, "Take it; this is my **body**."

Romans 9:8

In other words, it is not the children by **physical** descent who are God's children, but it is the children of the promise who are regarded as Abraham's offspring.

James 2:16

If one of you says to them, "Go in peace; keep warm and well fed," but does nothing about their physical needs, what good is it?

Mind

Numbers 23:19

God is not human, that he should lie, not a human being, that he should change his **mind**. Does he speak and then not act? Does he promise and not fulfill?

Deuteronomy 11:18

Fix these words of mine in your hearts and **mind**s; tie them as symbols on your hands and bind them on your foreheads.

Romans 8:5-6 [Full Chapter]

Those who live according to the flesh have their **mind**s set on what the flesh desires; but those who live in accordance with the Spirit have their **mind**s set on what the Spirit desires. The **mind** governed by the flesh is death, but the **mind** governed by the Spirit is life and peace.

Matthew 22:37

Jesus replied: "Love the Lord your God with all your heart and with all your soul and with all your **mind**."

Mark 8:33

But when Jesus turned and looked at his disciples, he rebuked Peter. "Get behind me, Satan!" he said. "You do not have in **mind** the concerns of God, but merely human concerns."

Mark 12:30

Love the Lord your God with all your heart and with all your soul and with all your **mind** and with all your strength.

John 15:18

If the world hates you, keep in **mind** that it hated me first.

Acts 15:24

We have heard that some went out from us without our authorization and disturbed you, troubling your **mind**s by what they said.

Romans 7:23

But I see another law at work in me, waging war against the law of my **mind** and making me a prisoner of the law of sin at work within me.

SPIRIT

John 16:13

But when he, the **Spirit** of truth, comes, he will guide you into all the truth. He will not speak on his own; he will speak only what he hears, and he will tell you what is yet to come.

Genesis 41:38

So Pharaoh asked them, "Can we find anyone like this man, one in whom is the **spirit** of God?"

Leviticus 19:31

Do not turn to mediums or seek out **spirit**ists, for you will be defiled by them. I am the Lord your God.

Deuteronomy 34:9

Now Joshua son of Nun was filled with the **spirit** of wisdom because Moses had laid his hands on him. So the Israelites listened to him and did what the Lord had commanded Moses.

Matthew 3:11

I baptize you with water for repentance. But after me comes one who is more powerful than I, whose sandals I am not worthy to carry. He will baptize you with the Holy **Spirit** and fire.

Matthew 3:16

As soon as Jesus was baptized, he went up out of the water. At that moment heaven was opened, and he saw the **Spirit** of God descending like a dove and alighting on him.

Matthew 5:3

Blessed are the poor in **spirit**, for theirs is the kingdom of heaven.

Matthew 10:20

For it will not be you speaking, but the **Spirit** of your Father speaking through you.

Matthew 12:18

Here is my servant whom I have chosen, the one I love, in whom I delight; I will put my **Spirit** on him, and he will proclaim justice to the nations.

Matthew 12:31

And so I tell you, every kind of sin and slander can be forgiven, but blasphemy against the **Spirit** will not be forgiven.

Matthew 27:50

And when Jesus had cried out again in a loud voice, he gave up his **spirit**.

Matthew 28:19

Therefore go and make disciples of all nations, baptizing them in the name of the Father and of the Son and of the Holy **Spirit**,

Mark 1:10

Just as Jesus was coming up out of the water, he saw heaven being torn open and the **Spirit** descending on him like a dove.

Romans 1:11

I long to see you so that I may impart to you some **spirit**ual gift to make you strong—

Romans 5:5

And hope does not put us to shame, because God's love has been poured out into our hearts through the Holy **Spirit**, who has been given to us.

Romans 8:6

The mind governed by the flesh is death, but the mind governed by the **Spirit** is life and peace.

Romans 8:14

For those who are led by the **Spirit** of God are the children of God.

Romans 12:11

Never be lacking in zeal, but keep your **spirit**ual fervor, serving the Lord.

1 Corinthians 2:12

What we have received is not the **spirit** of the world, but the **Spirit** who is from God, so that we may understand what God has freely given us.

1 Corinthians 3:16

Don't you know that you yourselves are God's temple and that God's **Spirit** dwells in your midst?

1 Corinthians 6:17

But whoever is united with the Lord is one with him in **spirit**.

Ephesians 1:17

I keep asking that the God of our Lord Jesus Christ, the glorious Father, may give you the **Spirit** of wisdom and revelation, so that you may know him better.

Ephesians 2:22

And in him you too are being built together to become a dwelling in which God lives by his **Spirit**.

Ephesians 3:16

I pray that out of his glorious riches he may strengthen you with power through his **Spirit** in your inner being,

Ephesians 4:4

There is one body and one **Spirit**, just as you were called to one hope when you were called.

Philippians 2:2

Then make my joy complete by being like-minded, having the same love, being one in **spirit** and of one mind.

Philippians 4:23

The grace of the Lord Jesus Christ be with your **spirit**. Amen.

Revelation 4:5

From the throne came flashes of lightning, rumblings and peals of thunder. In front of the throne, seven lamps were blazing. These are the seven **spirit**s of God.

1 Peter 3:4

Rather, it should be that of your inner self, the unfading beauty of a gentle and quiet **spirit**, which is of great worth in God's sight.

1 Peter 2:2

Like newborn babies, crave pure **spirit**ual milk, so that by it you may grow up in your salvation.

Hebrews 4:12

For the word of God is alive and active. Sharper than any double-edged sword, it penetrates even to dividing soul and **spirit**, joints and marrow; it judges the thoughts and attitudes of the heart.

Hebrews 1:14

Are not all angels ministering **spirit**s sent to serve those who will inherit salvation?

John 16:13

But when he, the **Spirit** of **truth**, comes, he will guide you into all the **truth**. He will not speak on his own; he will speak only what he hears, **and** he will tell you what is yet to come.

John 14:17

The Spirit of truth. The world cannot accept him, because it neither sees him nor knows him. But you know him, for he lives with you and will be in you.

Ephesians 1:13

And you also were included in Christ when you heard the message of truth, the gospel of your salvation.

When you believed, you were marked in him with a seal, the promised Holy Spirit.

Affliction & Suffering

2 Corinthians 4:17

For our light and momentary troubles are achieving for us an eternal glory that far outweighs them all.

Romans 12:12

Be joyful in hope, patient in **affliction**, faithful in prayer.

Isaiah 48:10

See, I have refined you, though not as silver; I have tested you in the furnace of **affliction**.

Job 36:15

But those who suffer he delivers in their suffering; he speaks to them in their **affliction**.

Job 36:21

Beware of turning to evil, which you seem to prefer to **affliction**.

Psalm 25:18

Look on my **affliction** and my distress and take away all my sins.

Psalm 31:7

I will be glad and rejoice in your love, for you saw my **affliction** and knew the anguish of my soul.

Psalm 107:41

But he lifted the needy out of their **affliction** and increased their families like flocks.

Genesis 41:52

The second son he named Ephraim and said, "It is because God has made me fruitful in the land of my **suffering**."

Job 2:13

Then they sat on the ground with him for seven days and seven nights. No one said a word to him, because they saw how great his **suffering** was.

Psalm 22:24

For he has not despised or scorned the **suffering** of the afflicted one; he has not hidden his face from him but has listened to his cry for help.

Psalm 119:50

My comfort in my **suffering** is this: Your promise preserves my life.

Isaiah 52:13

See, my servant will act wisely; he will be raised and lifted up and highly exalted.

Mark 5:34

He said to her, "Daughter, your faith has healed you. Go in peace and be freed from your **suffering**."

Acts 5:41

The apostles left the Sanhedrin, rejoicing because they had been counted worthy of **suffering** disgrace for the Name.

Romans 8:17

Now if we are children, then we are heirs—heirs of God and co-heirs with Christ, if indeed we share in his **suffering**s in order that we may also share in his glory.

Romans 8:18

I consider that our present **suffering**s are not worth comparing with the glory that will be revealed in us.

2 Corinthians 1:7

And our hope for you is firm, because we know that just as you share in our **suffering**s, so also you share in our comfort.

Ephesians 3:13

I ask you, therefore, not to be discouraged because of my **suffering**s for you, which are your glory.

1 Thessalonians 1:6

You became imitators of us and of the Lord, for you welcomed the message in the midst of severe **suffering** with the joy given by the Holy Spirit.

2 Timothy 1:8

So do not be ashamed of the testimony about our Lord or of me his prisoner. Rather, join with me in **suffering** for the gospel, by the power of God.

Author Biographies

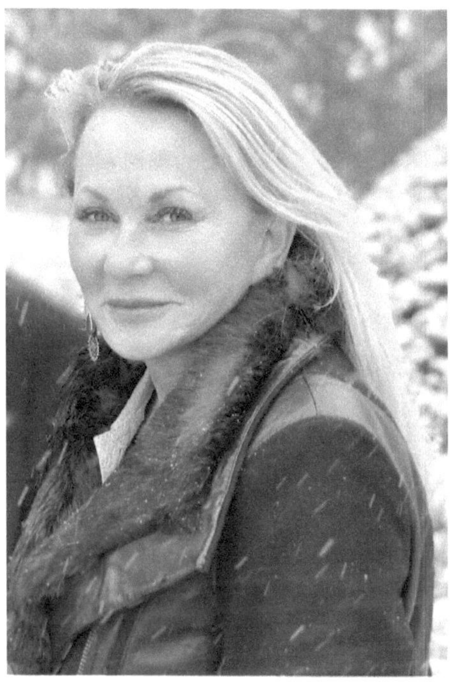

Kim Alumbaugh, M.D.

Board-certified Obstetrician/Gynecologist … practicing 20 years in Louisville, KY. She is one of the founders of Total Woman, the first Ob/Gyn Medical spa providing medical and in-office surgical care as well as ancillary services like physical therapy, massage and cosmetic enhancement. She and her husband Daniel Varga, MD have four amazing children, a fantastic son-in-law, and the perfect grandchild. Dr. Alumbaugh feels incredibly blessed to have "welcomed to the world" more than 5,000 babies.

***

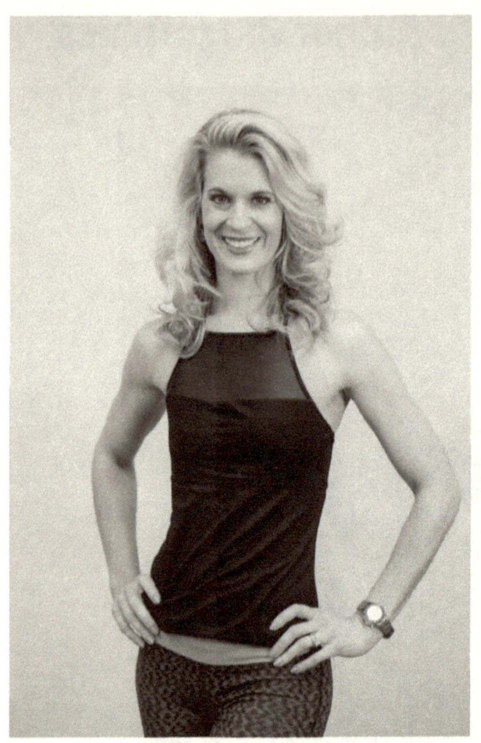

Alison Cardoza

ACSM Certified Personal Trainer and Fitour Group Exercise Instructor. She has over 15 years experience working with Baptist Health Milestone Wellness Center in both of those capacities.

As a former NFL Cheerleader, Alison enjoys teaching dance and cheer choreography to clients.

Alison is a wife to John and a mother to Alexa.

***

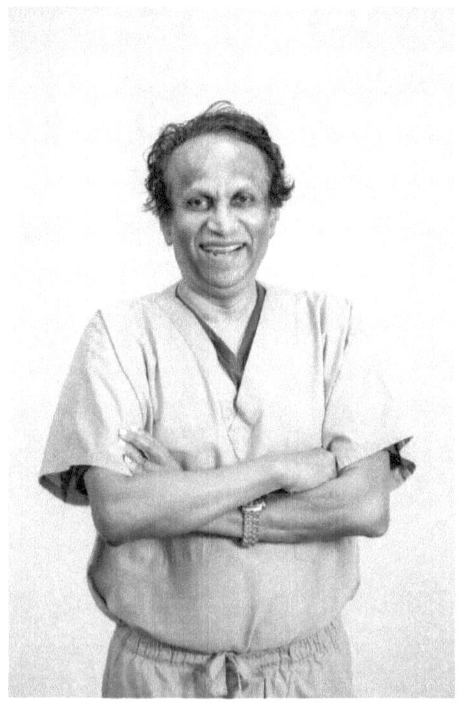

Ponnattu K. Cherian, M.D.

PK Cherian, M.D. is a board certified Cardiologist practicing in Louisville KY for 40 years.

10+ years, with Norton Heart Specialists, the largest Cardiology group in Louisville.

His wife of 47 years is Dr. Saramma Cherian. Together they have raised one son, Prasad and a daughter, Priya Cherian Huskins.

***

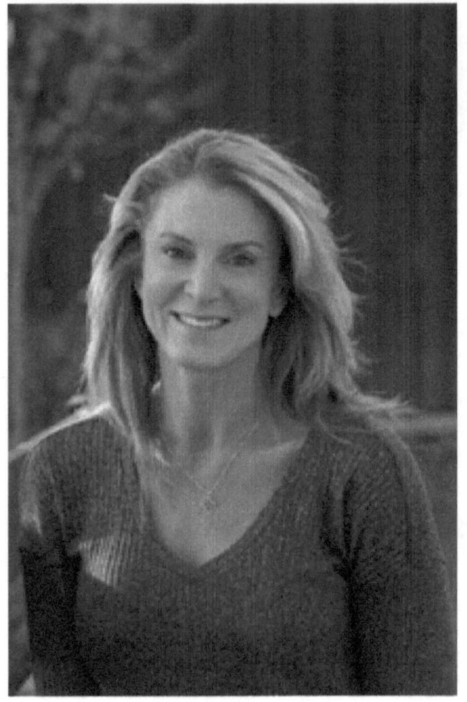

Jennifer DeGrella

Group fitness instructor and Personal trainer.

ACE certified since 1990, with special emphasis on TRX training.

Except for a three–year tenure with another health club, Jennifer has been employed by Baptist Health Milestone Wellness Center since 1997.

Single with 4 beautiful daughters.

***

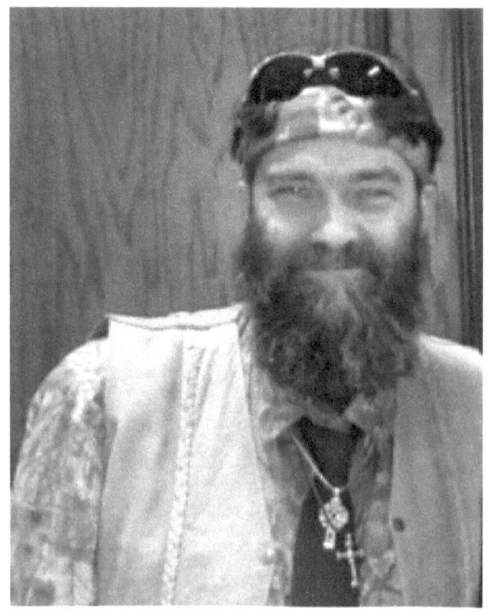

Phil Drake

Pastor for ten years before becoming a professional Life Coach.

Masters degree in Clinical Mental Health Counseling.

Graduate certificate in Addictions Counseling.

Married for 40 years, with one adult child.

***

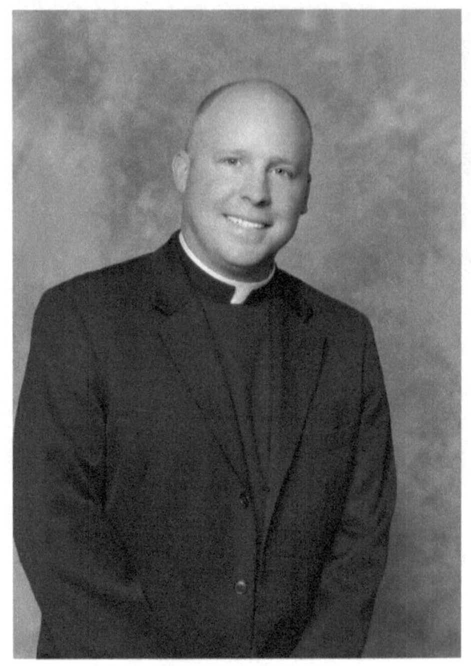

Rev. Father Shayne R. Duvall

Priest of the Archdiocese of Louisville,

Pastor of St. Raphael the Archangel Catholic Church in Louisville, KY.

Graduate of the University of Louisville with Bachelor of Science Degree in Justice Administration.

Graduate of Saint Meinrad Seminary and School of Theology, with Master of Divinity and Master of Theological Studies.

***

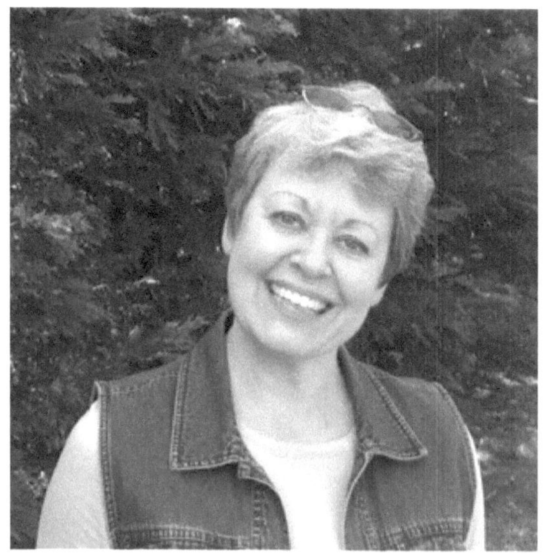

Mary Gaskins

Registered Dietitian Nutritionist.

Certified Diabetes Educator.

Member of Louisville Christian Writers.

Former Coordinator of Kentucky Christian Writers Conference.

Married, mother, grandmother.

***

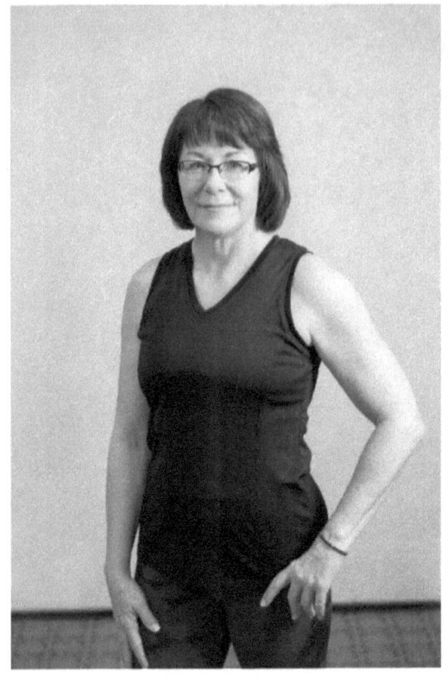

Mary M. Hayes

ACSM Certified Personal Trainer.

ACE Orthopedic Exercise Specialist.

16 years experience at Baptist Health Milestone Wellness Center in both capacities.

Proud mother of two and grandmother of one.

***

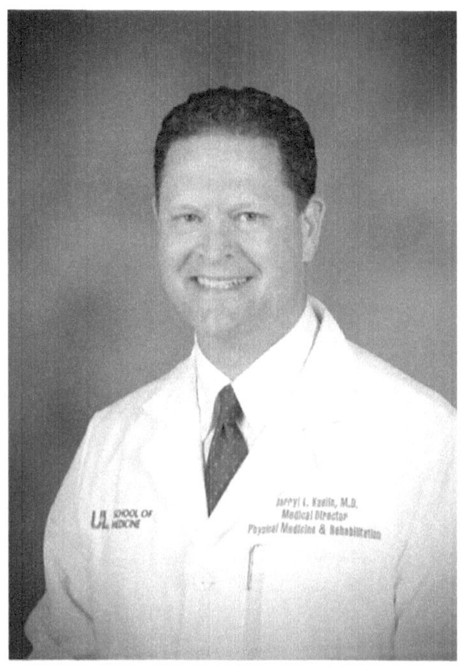

Darryl Kaelin, M.D.

Professor and University of Louisville Endowed Chair of Stroke and Brain Injury Rehabilitation.

Medical Director of the Frazier Rehabilitation Institute.

Chief of the Division of Physical Medicine and Rehabilitation in UL Department of Neurological Surgery.

Dr. Kaelin and his wife, Brenna, have been married since 1991 with three children, Audrey, Austin and Adam.

***

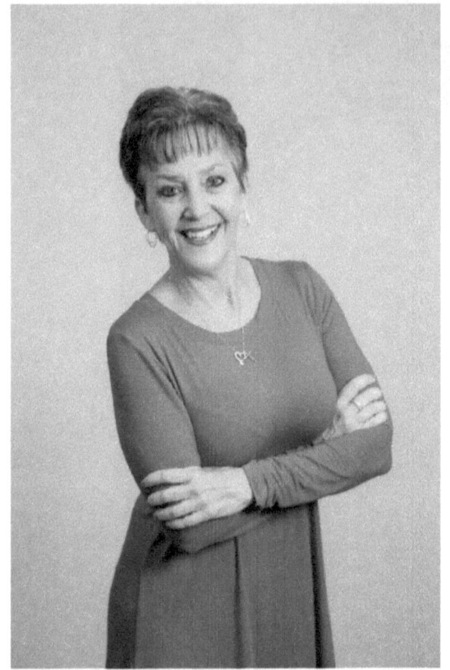

Elizabeth B. Lewis

Life Coach/Relationship Coach/Author/Speaker.

Author of *First Date Next Mate: Perspectives in Dating the "Next" Time Around.*

President of Love and Laughter Life Coaching, LLC www.loveandlaughterlifecoaching.com

Founder/President of Singles Meet Singles, LLC.

Retired Elementary Teacher- 27 years.

Elder at Middletown Christian Church. Widow with 2 adult children.

***

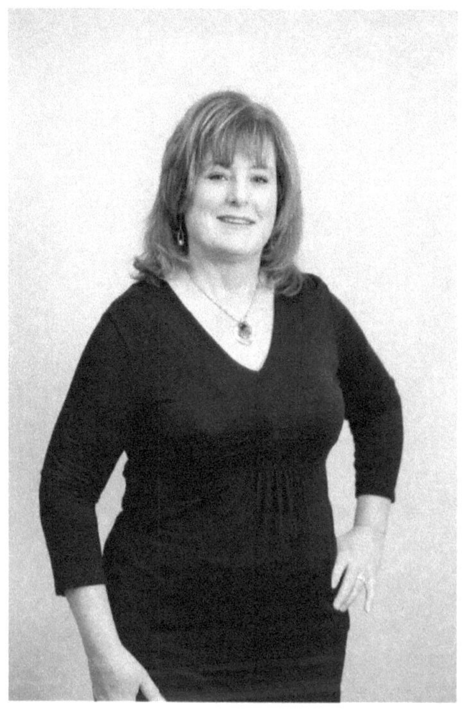

Dena Mullin

30 years as a Physical Therapist, earning her doctorate in 2016.

Special PT interests include foot and ankle biomechanics, osteoporosis education, Kinesio taping, and sports medicine.

Employed by Baptist Health Milestone Wellness Center for 15+ years.

Married for 20 years to Michael Mullin with one 15 year old daughter and two Shih Tzus.

***

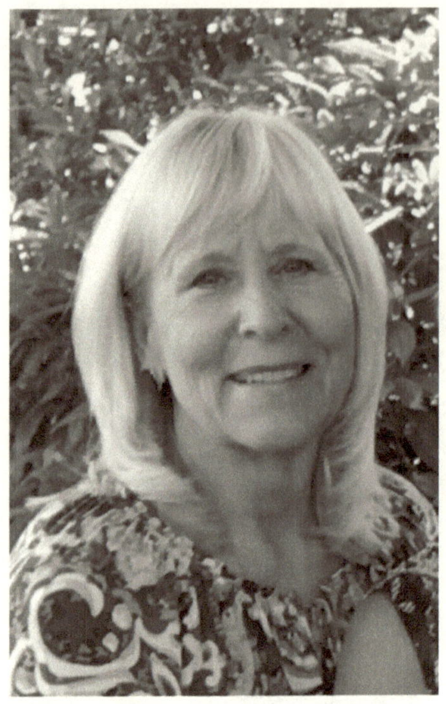

Nancy Ogle

Bible Study Fellowship Teaching Leader for 24 years.

Resides in Crestwood, Kentucky.

Married to Bruce for 40 years.

Mom to two adult and married children, Lauren and Eric.

Grandma to Sam, age 4; and Cora, age 1.

***

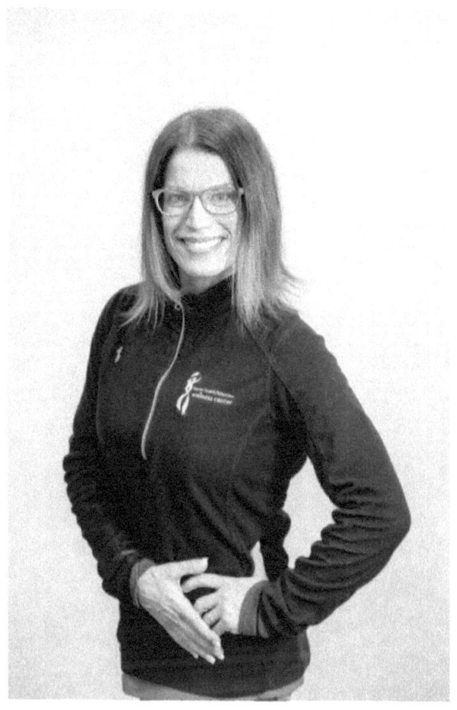

Bekki Jo Tressler

27 years as a fitness professional, including beginner/intermediate/advanced machine and mat based Pilates, AFAA Certified Personal Trainer, yoga, barre and cycling.

Joined fitness staff at Baptist Milestone in 1997.

Teaches college level Sociology in her spare time.

Married to Wayne with three great kids and one grandchild on the way.

***

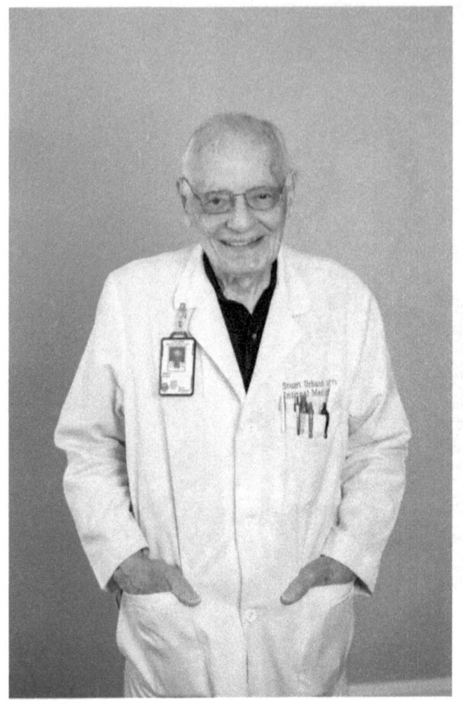

Stuart Urbach, MD

Board certified in Internal Medicine.

University of Louisville Associate Clinical Professor of Medicine.

Private practice, Louisville, KY for 63 years.

Married to the late Sherri Urbach for 60 years.

One son, two daughters and three beautiful granddaughters.

***

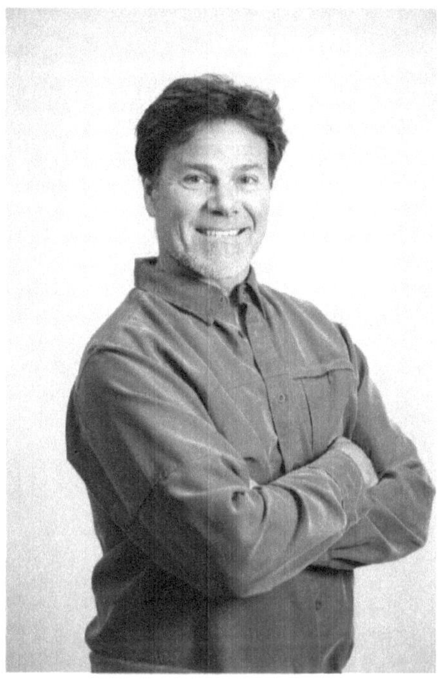

Zorre' Z. Kimura, PT, DPT

Physical Therapist at Baptist Health Milestone Wellness Center. APTA Credentialed Clinical Instructor. Adjunct Professor, PT Doctorate Program at Bellarmine University.Treatment approaches featuring dry needling, soft tissue mobilization, and aquatic therapy.

1982 Graduate of Saint Louis University PT Program with a doctorate in Physical Therapy from Evidence in Motion.

Enjoys being on the water whenever he can via boat, paddle board, or Catamaran. Happily married and has two awesome daughters.

***

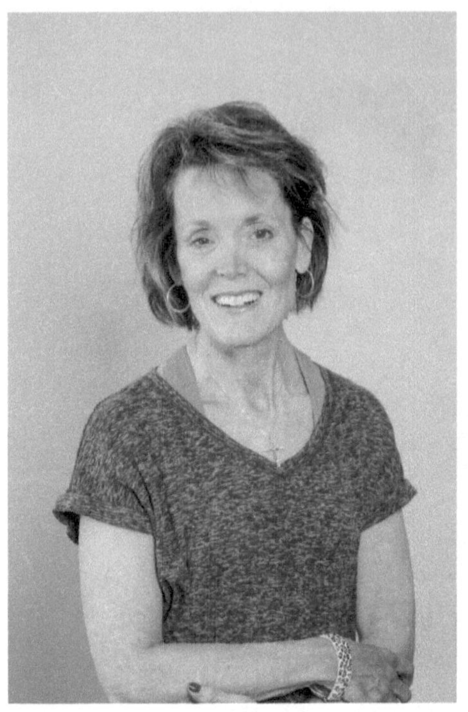

Mary Varga

Author of *The Light Through My Tunnel*. Founder and owner SilverStrength® serving Seniors in Louisville, KY since 2010. ACSM Certified Personal Trainer. Fitour Certified Senior Group Fitness Instructor.

Single with one adult son, Andrew Daugherty.

Survivor of Traumatic Brain Injury (TBI) in 1997.

Member of Louisville Christian Writers (LCW).

Attends Weekly Bible Study at Bible Study Fellowship (BSF).

***